Dr. Lendon Smith's

DIET PLAN
for
TEENAGERS

BOOKS BY LENDON SMITH, M.D.

Dr. Lendon Smith's

DIET PLAN
for
TEENAGERS

LENDON SMITH, M.D.
with Martha Rose Shulman

McGraw-Hill Book Company
New York St. Louis San Francisco Bogotá Hamburg
Johannesburg London Madrid Mexico Milan Montreal
New Delhi Panama Paris São Paulo Singapore
Sydney Tokyo Toronto

1 2 3 4 5 6 7 8 9 A G A G 8 7

First paperback edition, 1987.

ISBN 0-07-058700-0 (H.C.)

ISBN 0-07-058706-X (PBK.)

LIBRARY OF CONGRESS CATALOGING-IN-PUBLICATION DATA

Smith, Lendon H., 1921–
   Dr. Lendon Smith's diet plan for teenagers.
   1. Youth—Nutrition. I. Shulman, Martha Rose.
II. Title. III. Title: Diet plan for teenagers.
[DNLM: 1. Diet—in adolescence. QT 235 S654d]
RJ235.S55   1986   613.2'088055   85-24194
ISBN 0-07-058700-0 (h.c.)

ISBN 0-07-058706-X (pbk.)

BOOK DESIGN BY PATRICE FODERO

I would like to dedicate this book to my dear wife, Julie. She is still with me and feeding me and holding me together. Her foods keep me as lusty and vigorous as a healthy adolescent.

Preface: What Can I Eat?

This book is for those teenagers who are dissatisfied with the size and shape of their bodies. It is designed to give teenagers the feeling that they can exercise some kind of control over their lives and bodies, by helping them understand their bodies and showing them that the way they feel, look, and think at different times is directly related to the way they feel about themselves. As you adolescents learn to read your body, you will begin to accept it more, because you will see that with proper diet and exercise you can control some of the things that are happening to it. You may not be able to control the fact that your breasts are growing, but you can get them to stop hurting so much and prevent that bloated "fat" feeling before your periods by altering your diet. You might find that a food allergy is giving you those nosebleeds, or that the fast food you eat every day is responsible for your acne. Other teenage problems, both physical and mental (bad breath, stomachaches, headaches, depression), can be aided with a dietary approach. Balance the body and it will be less susceptible to acne, mono, fatigue, and insomnia. Once you become aware of some basic physiological and nutritional facts, you will learn to read body clues that indicate that a tilt has occurred, and you will know what will bring the body back into balance.

TO THE TEENAGER: We hope in this book to make you realize that you are not alone. We adults had to go through all the
stresses and pains and frustrations that you are going through.
You are growing, you are changing, you are maturing, and you
are still expected to take care of yourself, get your studies done,
and be cheerful. You are terribly hungry, and yet, if you are a
girl, you are plagued by the "if you're thin, you're in" standard,
and you will suffer from an interminable conflict with food,
which could lead you to bulimia or anorexia.

If you are a boy you may be discouraged that your legs are
heavy and your chest looks caved in no matter how much you
eat. You can't seem to make muscles out of your food.

With this book, food and diet will cease to be a mystery to
you, for we will unravel the simple mechanics of nutrition and
digestion. Exercise will begin to take on a new importance as
you use it to replace deprivation and starvation and fad diets as a
means of weight control. You will learn how to eat to get the best
possible performance from your particular body—in school and
in sports. With this new understanding of yourself and your
body, the menus and recipes we will provide herein will make
perfect sense to you, and they should make your mouth water.

TO THE PARENT: As I travel about the country and speak at
PTA meetings, dental conferences, and health and fitness
shows, I am overwhelmed by the questions asked about the
teenage diet. The parents want the best for their youngsters, but
all their children want to eat are hamburgers, fries, and soft
drinks.

The food that Martha Rose Shulman presents in this book
will please the entire family. Parents and kids will reap the
benefits of her delicious, easy-to-prepare meals. Teenagers will
be amazed to find that some of these foods will even taste like
their favorite high-fat, high-salt and high-sugar junk food! You
will be startled to find that many of the foods you thought were
forbidden, like bread, pizza, spaghetti, and ice cream, are allowed if made with whole, low-fat ingredients, or sweetened
with fruit rather than sugar.

There is more than one way to make a milkshake, and Martha Rose knows the low-calorie, high-nutrition ways. Sugar, salt,

fat, and meat can all be reduced or substituted for by foods that stop the physiological cravings, and half the time your children will never even know it's happening. And, as you'll see from the nutrient key to each recipe, they'll be getting the best foods for them. And contrary to popular belief, eating well does not require extra time.

I hope that you and your children will find some answers here. We can't smooth out all the problems that come up during these confusing adolescent years, but we can get these teenagers into such good shape that they can cope with things more easily.

Acknowledgments

My sincere thanks to my dear friend and nutrition information supplier, Anne Condas. She is the spark behind the B.E.A.N.S. (Better Education and Nutritional Snacks) program in the central California area and is spreading the word about nutritional food.

Nancy Hoffman has been of great help with the manuscript. She has reduced the numbers of redundancies and non sequiturs. Peggy Moss was helpful in guiding and directing the manuscript in its early stages.

Contents

Introduction: Feeding the Adolescent

TO THE TEENAGER: I was an adolescent once. And I am relieved that I do not have to go through that age again. It was miserable and exciting, anxious anticipation alternating with crashing boredom, heady optimism slipping into paralyzing depression. It was acute awareness of bodily changes over which I had no control. What was going on? Who could I talk to? There were sudden hungers that seemed insatiable, and feelings of skepticism, suspicion, and outright paranoia: Did my friends talk about me behind my back? Was I the only one with these strange thoughts and urges? Was I normal? I got good grades at school, but they made me the joke editor of the class paper. Were they laughing at me or with me?

My hips, thighs, and buttocks seemed too big at age fourteen. My shoulders sloped and did not match the lower parts of me. It took me about three years to become more proportional and then to acquire (and still to have) only twenty-two hairs on my chest. I can remember how overjoyed I was at age sixteen when someone called me "Hey, slim." And I had always thought of myself as gross and ungainly.

I don't think I have ever met an adolescent—while growing up or in my practice—who really liked the package he or she came in. Some felt they were too fat, some too thin, some too tall, others too short. It is true—some were at the extremes of "normal." But humans come in all colors, sizes, and shapes, largely determined by their hereditary. Some had thick ankles; some were knock-kneed while others were bowlegged. Some girls had breasts they thought were too large or pendulous, while the others had breasts that for them were too small. A few had three; abnormal, but not unheard-of.

Probably the best word for defining the way adolescents perceive their relationship with their bodies is "trapped." This goes along with their overall life view. "What's the point? Why was I born? Nothing is fair. No one listens to my side of any story. It's up at seven, eat, school, chores, homework, eat, and bed. I'd like to have a little fun." Everything seems to be preordained ("Why did I have to inherit my mother's stupid body?") or illegal ("I'd like to run away, smoke pot, and be free as a bird") or immoral ("I wish I could have a baby, be independent, and find my own way").

In fact, there are some things that really are *not* fair. One is the fashion-model image that Madison Avenue and Hollywood relentlessly place in front of teenage eyes, so that girls, in particular, are brainwashed into thinking that this is the only way to look, that these kinds of looks are all that count, that a skinny body and a skinny body alone will assure popularity and success.

Another, paradoxically, is the food with which the junk food and fast food industries have so successfully flooded our country. The very foods so appealing to teenagers, largely because Mom is too busy to cook and their local hangouts are now shopping malls where fast food establishments abound, are the foods that contain too much fat, too much salt, too much sugar, and too much meat. A slim, trim figure is hard to maintain if this type of food is eaten consistently. It was bad enough when I was young and we would stuff our faces with cherry cokes, French fries, and ice cream sodas. Now the ice cream sodas and shakes aren't even made with dairy products, and teenagers have a much wider choice of high-calorie fast foods, from pizzas to croissant sandwiches to Big Macs to Kentucky Fried Chicken. Some of the greasy hamburgers on white buns are called, appropriately, "belly bombers." And these days the Cokes, shakes, and hamburgers are twice as big as they used to be.

Teenagers are not eating properly, and this lopsided nutritional intake is making some of them fat, some of them mean, and, if they survive this phase, many of them grow up to be saddled with obesity, diabetes, frequent infections, insomnia, hypertension, heart attacks, surliness, low energy, and, to top it all off, osteoporosis.

And *we* thought we were the best-fed people in the world. We are just the *most* fed.

TO THE PARENT: Most teenagers have a very tenuous self-image. This is certainly understandable, for their bodies are changing daily, growing in ways that are scary and distasteful to many. Muscles, glands, and fat pads spring up overnight; weight and girth fluctuate. New hormones are at work, and kids cannot tell from one day to the next if their complexions will be free of pimples, if their stomachs will be bloated, or if they will feel depressed or breezy.

While nothing else in life seems to be certain, the Hollywood image of beauty remains a constant. So it is not surprising that teenage girls latch onto this as a personal goal and become obsessed with dieting and irrational in their desire to be skinny. They all want to be at least 5 pounds lighter. The typical teenage girl believes that no boy would ever look at her if she didn't have a model's body. The fact that all body types are different, that some people are not meant to be thin models in bathing suits on the cover of *Vogue,* is lost on her. She doesn't want to hear about different body types; she is so obsessed with looking at herself in the mirror that she doesn't notice that flesh hangs differently on various types of bodies. At a time when most things seem to be out of control, her weight becomes something she thinks she might be able to control. In the extreme she may become anorectic or bulimic, conditions which are becoming epidemic in our country.

The problem is that it is nearly impossible to have any real control over one's weight when one knows very little about food, and when most of the foods waved in front of one's eyes are high in excess, empty calories. So it's not surprising that almost everyone is confused about eating, that 10 percent of the nation's adolescents are obese and a large percent are overweight. This is particularly unfortunate because overeating in teenage years can result in a lifetime of weight problems. Adolescents are still manufacturing fat cells. On the other hand, not getting enough nutrients during the teenage years can result in health problems later on in life, including complications in childbearing and lactation.

Yet teenagers must eat. They are always hungry because they are going through a dramatic growth spurt, and their need for calories and nutrients is very high. Boys, who are adding on more lean body tissue (muscle and bone) than soft body tissue, are not as concerned with dieting as girls. But girls have the same hunger, perhaps not quite as strong, and they need as much calcium, manganese, magnesium, molybdenum, zinc, phosphorus, iodine, vitamins, and other minerals as do the adolescent boys. How do they obtain these same nutrients from at least 20 percent fewer calories? Not so easy, considering their junk food diets.

But teenagers won't change their eating habits unless they see some real advantage in doing so. They must see the connection between the way they look and feel and what they eat before they will make any alterations. They must begin to understand why the key to weight loss and maintenance is *not dieting, but eating the right foods*. And the "right foods" have to taste good and be familiar. When they and their parents have begun to acquire knowledge about what they eat, and about their bodies, they will no longer be at war with food (and with each other), and instead they will be able to make intelligent decisions about how they are going to feed themselves.

Parents can help their teenage children in this struggle not just by emptying the kitchen of junk food and using the menu plans in this book, but by better understanding the psychological nature of their children's dietary problems. It's easy and normal to become exasperated with adolescents; will they ever grow out of their self-involved funk? Constantly we, their parents, must remind ourselves that we were teenagers once too, and we must remember back to that time when so many things frightened or confused us.

We all have an image of ourselves, good or bad, and it is largely determined by how accepting our parents or caretakers were. If we got good strokes as little babies, we have mentally filed all that goodness away in some way. We may have temporary setbacks as we march through life, but we will never be completely destroyed because there is that glowing ember deep in our psyche, saying "You're okay." During the teenage years the ember may become dim, and the need for approval from parents and acceptance by peers becomes overwhelming.

If youngsters cannot find acceptance, stress shows up, and one way they might cope with it is by eating. Or by starving themselves. Or by bingeing followed by self-induced vomiting or laxative-controlled diarrhea. Or the body may show up with a psychosomatic problem: acne breaks out, or the palms may become sweaty all the time, or stuttering begins.

Psychiatrists tell us that the struggling adolescent is being torn between a drive for independence and the need for dependence on parents and caretakers. Why does it take so long to grow up? What do parents do with adolescents while waiting for them to grow up? What do teenagers do with themselves while waiting to be old enough to join the army, finish school, go to college, start a family, or get a job? Study, do the chores, stare into space, go to the movies, hang out at the shopping mall, talk with friends, neck, make out, pout or be passive-aggressive with adults. In short, they try to get some control over their lives.

If all the avenues of independence and autonomy are closed to teenagers, they may find that controlling some of their body functions may offer some feeling of power and independence that they lack. We all need to feel good about ourselves, and that delightful high of being able to say "I'm in charge," should be present daily. Some can do it with sports or music or academic skills. Others have a harder time finding something that is "theirs," and these are the ones who are more susceptible to eating disorders, although overachievers, ironically, seem to be susceptible also.

Even with more understanding, psychological and physiological, the problem of changing teenage eating habits remains. Many well-meaning parents believe that if the food is on the grocery store shelves it must be all right to eat. Parents claim that they have no time to cook and feed their kids a proper meal, and if they do find the time to fix one, the surly youth will not eat it.

What makes the problem even greater today than it was when I began my medical practice over 35 years ago, is that the structure of the American family has changed. Most mothers are now in the work force, and can spend far less time than they used to in the kitchen; no longer can they turn out three square meals a day for their children and husbands; but since they're often still unfairly expected to do so, they must often cut corners with convenience foods. They are not there when their children, now carrying their own keys, come home from school, hungry for a snack—or, in later years when there are more after-school commitments, starving for dinner. And husbands, if they are present, have not learned, or have not been willing to learn, to lend a hand in meal planning and cooking for the family. Because this development is a relatively recent one in our society, many families have become disorganized about their eating, so the quality of their diet has declined.

I have witnessed a kind of anxiety among children and teenagers that I believe exists because the source and nature of their next meal is not the certainty it used to be. It is a "What can I eat?" anxiety that disappears when regular meals and snacks can be counted on. Because of the constant, great demands of the growing body during adolescence, it makes sense that eating should be a preoccupation. Add to the biological demands the mixed messages that (a) the teen should be thin and that (b) junk food will make him and her happy; couple all this with the fact that the food one is eating probably affects the blood sugar and the ability to reason, and it's no wonder anxiety about eating becomes so exaggerated. Teenagers already have racing hormones to deal with and then here comes general malaise and ennui, the fear of the bodily changes that are occurring (which might be associated with eating in the subconscious mind), paranoia, and dissatisfaction with parental rules and the world at large. Isn't that enough?

The only solution to the eating problem is to develop a new approach, to develop new systems, so that even if families are not sitting down together around a table every morning and night, they are still eating regular, balanced meals. Teenagers can get involved, and the process can be fun, and certainly tasty. Menu organization and healthy snack planning and food preparation are things that teenagers can do with their families or together in groups, or even while watching television. It's easy to chat and gossip while chopping vegetables, and, with a suitable headpiece, they can even prepare food while on the phone.

Being more involved in feeding themselves will give teenagers a new sense of independence and a positive kind of control over their bodies. Right now it is in their nature to feel that their lives are filled with drudgery, and that the easiest way to feed themselves is by eating Kentucky Fried Chicken, burgers and fries, and pizzas. So what if this makes them surly and gives them oily skin—they taste good. The problem with that is, those very feelings of drudgery and despair are brought on in part by all the excess sugar and fat in the junk food. Biochemically the kids don't stand a chance when they eat these foods. Their lives become an endless cycle of starvation and bingeing, of losing weight and gaining it back, of depression and exhaustion and the secondary effects on the thyroid, the brain, and the intestinal tract. This is a cycle that begins and ends in tears and feelings of loss of control.

We can regain that power by learning how to nourish ourselves. Contrary to popular belief, "diets" do not teach control. They just put us in an unnatural state of semistarvation. They're depressing to stay on because all they say is *"don't."* Anyway, most end up going *off* the diets, hating themselves and getting even more depressed. It's a no-win situation.

So give our approach a try. It is safe and natural. So many teens feel there is no way out of the entrapment of their age, in a body they did not want to inherit and in a city and a school and a neighborhood that they feel are the pits. With the diet herein described, the teen should be able to feel some sense of control over his or her daily life. We think it will help teenagers make a little sense out of these difficult years.

CHAPTER 1

What Is Thin Anyway?

Most young people have a very confused self-image, and the picture they would like to have of their bodies usually bears little resemblance to what their bodies actually look like. Studies have shown that up to 60 percent of teenage girls in the *normal* weight range view themselves as overweight. (Boys, on the other hand, often think of themselves as underweight.) It seems logical that if a young, maturing female looks at the magazine cover of *Vogue, Harper's Bazaar, Mademoiselle, Cosmopolitan,* or *Glamour* and then looks in the mirror, she is going to assume that she has to lose some weight. The fashion and advertising industries promote an image that is rail-thin. The message is that it's only possible to be happy and successful if you are *thin*, almost prepubertal, and this standard has resulted in an obsession among women that starts in adolescence, a very trying time.

It is a time of stress and violent change anyway, and then to be saddled with a body that is less than perfect (not thin), and to have to live in that body the rest of one's life, well, is discouraging to say the least. A little girl becomes a woman in just a few short years and develops those curves which nature says she is supposed to have—even if Yves St. Laurent and Madison Avenue don't agree. She may look on these normal curves and appropriate fat pads as a sign of pathological obesity which requires extreme measures now.

The emphasis on skinny is so strong in our culture that it is practically impossible for women and men, especially the younger ones, to accept the fact that evolution has molded women with flesh. These fashion demands are very recent, a phenomenon of the twentieth century. Even as late as the turn of the century, a certain amount of fat was considered advantageous as a protection against diseases such as tuberculosis, dysentery, and typhoid fever, which were more likely to defeat the thin. Infectious diseases were thought to be more threatening to the scrawny ones, so avoirdupois was an advantage. Throughout the ages, up until the middle of the eighteenth century, most of the earth's people lived in constant jeopardy of famine (many still do). First when men were hunters and gatherers, then when they began to cultivate the earth and their agricultural systems would break down because of droughts, it was important for men and women to have fat stores, for during times of want these would be their only source of fuel.

When does normal become fat? We need a little extra to get through the cold winter. Most normal people gain a little in the winter months, but it may be they also exercise less. Some actually seem to be hibernating—their metabolism seems to slow down.

Heaviness in the adult male, until recently, suggested success. But comparable fullness in the female suggested to many a weakness, a lack of self-control. This attitude is often reinforced by the unthinking physician, who is still taught in medical school that obesity is always due to this equation: If more calories are consumed than the metabolism can use, weight gain is inevitable.

My years in practice have taught me to believe that if the parents are able to instill a reasonably good self-image in their children, those children, as adults, will be able to accept themselves as normal human beings and will not have to spend the rest of their days looking for perfection, trying to impress the internalized parent that we all carry with us through life.

We have to teach the budding female that human reproduction requires some fat. A woman must have some stores of adipose tissue in order to nourish her baby. Women will not menstruate unless they have about 20 percent of their body weight as fat. Their fat, in a sense, "advertises" their fertility. Most men know; they see the breasts and the hips and know the women with those endowments are ready to date. Men's muscles advertise their ability to provide.

Paintings dating from the fifteenth to the seventeenth centuries idealize women as fertile, reproductive creatures, with round bellies and wide hips. From about 1700 to about 1920, the women depicted in paintings have full bosoms and bottoms, and narrow waists; theirs is a maternal image. But since the 1920s fashion has opted for slim, sylphlike women who seem always on the run, doing things upwardly mobile, bright, quick, clever, and having fun. Perhaps this lithe image began as a symbol of the liberation women have begun to experience in this century; but now it has become a confining one.

Another thing to be aware of when dieting is that excessive exercise, dieting, and anorexia contribute to an alarming bone loss in young people resembling osteoporosis. This happens in young women especially due to a related drop in estrogen during dieting which then affects bone structure, causing them to become much more susceptible to fractures. So, beware!

Bone-thin women stop ovulating, as if Mother Nature did not want them to get pregnant at that time. Very active women such as dancers and athletes may have irregular periods or stop menstruating altogether. This is fairly common, but irregular periods or cessation is a clue that the physiology of the endocrine system needs to be investigated by a doctor. See your gynecologist.

TO THE TEENAGER: Look around your class or observe the variety of shapes and sizes of people walking by on the street. Some are long and thin, some are short and thin, some are tall and fat and some are muscular, big and tall, etc. There are all sorts of styles of size and weight out there and you must be realistic enough to figure out what sort of a body you have and be satisfied with it.

Do you have fat ankles, fat feet, fat hands, and short, fat, tapering fingers? Those are genetically determined and you must get used to them and accept them. You have probably noticed those traits in a parent or grandparent or other relatives. It also means you will never be thin and scrawny—you have big bones and muscles. But that does not mean you should let yourself go; you must eat using the ideas in this book so that you will look the best in the body you inherited. You are a mixture of endomorph and mesomorph types and have a different physiology. Your intestines are longer than those of your thin classmate who has thin lips, long thin fingers, and can eat anything (ectomorph). You have a very efficient intestinal tract with acres more absorptive area than your scrawny friend.

The obsession to attain thinness has resulted in many unhealthy diets. There is a phenomenon called the "thin/fat person." This is an individual of normal weight who is a compulsive dieter because she is totally absorbed with being fashionably slim.

I once had a normally proportioned, 5-foot 9-inch female patient who thought she was fat. (The world thought she was thin; she thought she was fat; therefore, thin/fat.) It was during the late 1960s, when everyone wanted to look like the 90-pound model, Twiggy. The only way to do that was to stop eating altogether—or that was the perception of many young ladies, including my patient. She tried it.

At one point her parents took her to France, where they stayed in three-star hotels. Despite the entreaties of her parents and the good smells coming from the kitchen, Andrea deprived herself of some of the best cooking in the world. By the time they got to the coastal town of Biarritz, Andrea was down to 100 pounds, just skin and bones; but she thought she looked terrific. Her parents were quite worried, of course, but couldn't get her to eat. Every night they would urge her to come with them to the fancy hotel restaurant for dinner, but Andrea would insist that she'd eaten a late lunch with her friends at the beach. It all came to a head one night when Andrea passed out cold in her parents' bedroom, just before they left for dinner. It scared her and her parents, and a large dinner was ordered immediately in the room. Her parents stood over her while she ate (willingly, I might add), and that was the last of her reckless dieting.

Andrea had missed anorexia by the skin of her fortunately still-good teeth, but others are not so lucky. The epidemic proportions of eating disorders today reflect the emotional toll our society is paying for the slim standard. Even those without actual eating disorders have become very confused, as they constantly diet, putting their bodies into a state of semistarvation which results in fatigue, increased obsession with food, depression, chilliness, poorer performance in school, constipation, anxiety, amenorrhea, and mental sluggishness. Hunger is often viewed as the enemy; eating causes guilt feelings, and a general confusion over body signals results. Teenagers often don't know when they're actually hungry, and this causes the kind of distress reflected in their strange eating behavior.

A common sequel to repeated fasts is a compensatory decrease in thyroid function. The thyroid hormone is responsible for the activation of the metabolism of every cell of the body; without this, the various functions of the body slow down. With continued decreases in caloric intake, the thyroid assumes that a famine is going on, and so, to conserve energy, it sets the metabolic rate a few degrees lower. Body temperature drops; the victim slows down. It is a little like hibernating. But when the caloric intake is increased, the thyroid does not squirt out more thyroid right away and the owner of this insulted body finds that weight will be added even on a less-than-1,000-calorie-a-day diet.

Losing the ability to respond to body signals can be dangerous in many ways. Sometimes the body becomes ill as a signal that it wants to rest and fast from junk food. (Life-threatening diseases are Mother Nature's way of getting people to slow down.) Many of us won't stop racing our engines and stuffing ourselves with empty foods until we feel so lousy we have to. We must stop being rude to our bodies. I got sick with the flu after a four-week stressful tour, flying to a new city every day. My body was nice enough to wait until I got home before it pulled the rug out from under my immune system.

If we are always compulsively dieting and not listening to our body's most basic and obvious signal, *hunger*, then we will miss the other, sometimes more urgent messages. This happened to a patient of mine who got a case of hepatitis that was probably much worse than it would have been had she been responding to the clues her body was sending her. She was unlucky, of course, to have come into contact with the virus, but she refused to stop running herself ragged with exercise and dieting, even when she began to feel ill.

The day before she was brought to my office she had swum a mile. By the time I saw her she could hardly move, she was so weak. The hepatitis was so severe that it took her about a year and half to really feel strong and healthy again. If she had been getting enough nutrients and had been able to read the signals telling her to slow down she would have known she was sick before she'd done her liver even more damage, and she would have been able to recover more quickly. (If I had seen her recently, I would have given her an intravenous injection of vitamin C and gotten her well in just a few days. We didn't know in those days how bad diets and fatigue can exhaust the immune system. The viruses are always around, but they only invade one if the immune system is not guarding the gates.)

Even while she was lying around, feeling lousy and depressed, she was terrified that she would get "fat" (she weighed but 98 pounds). She expressed these fears to her somewhat impatient sister, whose response—"Well, she died thin"—finally made her see the folly of her obsession.

I know of other teenage girls who, because they associate being thinner with being happier, more popular, and better loved by parents and peers, refuse to eat in front of families and friends because they are afraid that this will evoke comments about their weight. Others exercise frantically in the bedroom with the door locked, so that no family member will see them in a leotard. Some are so embarrassed to be seen naked in the locker room that they routinely skip PE class. Prepubertal boys at age 11 to 14 years are often so chagrined about the small size of their organs and the lack of pubic hair that they too may refuse PE in order to avoid taking a shower afterward.

The developing teenage body undergoes great changes in fat distribution, muscle growth, and figure development. The increase of the fat layer feeds the teenage females fear of becoming fat. Feelings about their bodies are so volatile at this age that the slightest comment—a father telling his daughter, "You'd have a perfect figure if you could just lose about ten pounds," or the wrestling coach telling a boy he won't make the team at that weight, or the ballet teacher commenting on a rounding belly—can ruin a person's self-image and send her or him into an endless cycle of unhealthy dieting. If, at the age of 13, your brothers referred to you as "The Crisco Kid—all the fat's in the can," then no matter what your rear end really looks like, you will always be saddled with that self-contempt. Parents and teachers should try to be more sensitive about this (brothers will always be a pain). And teenagers shouldn't let those PE instructors or coaches get away with making disparaging remarks. Any teacher or coach who is making the teenager feel "fat," should be avoided; one can always change coaches or switch sports. The adolescent has enough pressures to cope with as it is.

Another reason that it's difficult for teenagers to get a handle on their body image is that the cultural image of beauty contrasts greatly with the food their culture is offering. While the models are stick-thin, the foods they are promoting are full of empty calories. The fast food establishments that cater to teenagers offer food that, for the most part, is high in fat and sugar. (A Big Mac has 541 calories, and roughly a third of them are fat. If you have a coke with it you get another 150 calories, all quick sugar; a milk shake would take it up another 330 [vanilla] to 360 [chocolate].) Television advertising appeals to this age group, and many of the foods that the thin models are pushing are items like potato chips (fat) and sweets. It's not surprising, with these mixed messages constantly being shouted at them, that teenagers are confused.

Given these situations, teenagers and their parents must attack the problem. First teenagers have to consider what they are eating. The fact that a teenager may feel fat or actually be heavier than he or she should be may be related to the amount of exercise done per day, and the diet. If one lives on fast foods and junk, that is too much fat, sugar, and salt. The fat and sugar are difficult to burn, and the salt makes one feel fat because it causes the body to retain water.

There are all kinds of changes the teenager can make, and they are not necessarily difficult; nor will they require one to stay away from the hangouts where one normally goes with friends (see Chapters 4 and 10). One doesn't have to eat sprouts and carrot sticks the rest of one's life—and one shouldn't.

Parents too need to learn more about what they are feeding their children. I knew a young girl who developed a fat complex very early in life, and began dieting when she was nine years old. She was tired of being teased by her brothers, tired of losing at hopscotch. Her mother was a perpetual dieter who took Dexedrine every day, not knowing how dangerous that was. She thought it would be a good idea if her little girl learned at an early age what was "fattening" and what was "thinning." Sally learned to stop eating potatoes, bread, and desserts. She got skim instead of whole milk. She didn't snack on cookies, but on fruit. The problem was that her mother's knowledge of "dos" and "don'ts" was quite limited, about as bad as most doctors'.

While instilling in her daughter feelings of guilt about eating desserts, she fed her double portions of marbled red meat for dinner every night. She prided herself on the quality and quantity of the food she fed her children, and her children grew up thinking that it was normal and healthy to have two 3-inch-thick lamb chops on their plates at dinner, or two thick hamburgers on white buns with lots of sugary ketchup, or several slices of juicy, fatty roast beef with Yorkshire pudding. Parents didn't know back then about all the fat hidden in red meat. "But it makes it taste so good." Sally was allowed to eat as much salad as she wanted, but her mother didn't realize that the Russian dressing she glopped on the iceberg lettuce and tomatoes every night was nothing but fat (from the mayonnaise) and sugar (from the ketchup).

Every morning Sally's mother made her a big, hearty breakfast, since she knew what an important meal that was. She also knew a little bit about cholesterol, so she didn't serve eggs every day. But on the alternate days she laid out big bowls of refined, commercial brands of cereal with sugar and milk. And on cold winter mornings it might be bacon (fat), or instant Ralston with chocolate chips—and that's better than hot chocolate with marshmallows! No wonder Sally had such a hard time losing that little tummy that her brothers called the "three-ring circus."

Lunch was another glaring example of Sally's mother's good-will but caloric ignorance. Her sandwiches were made on white bread (enriched with nine added vitamins and minerals after the processors took 29 nutrients out of the flour) and usually consisted of mayonnaise and several slices of bologna and processed American cheese. These could have been called "refined fat, sandwiches."

Sally's diet was a paradox. She wasn't allowed to have candy bars or many Cokes, and rarely did she eat potato chips or Fritos; these foods just were not around. But her mother's ideas about good food were a haphazard mixture of what her own mother had cooked and what seemed to be quality. "Certainly, if those foods are advertised they must be good for us. The government checks on all those things, doesn't it? They wouldn't allow bad foods to be sold, would they?" Sally spent a miserable childhood, the butt of peer jokes because her mother fed her "good" food. Now as an adult she still carries her tarnished self-image though she was able to dump some of the unwanted pounds in adolescence.

TO THE TEENAGER: Understanding your body will help you comprehend why you sometimes feel "fat" and sluggish. You may be growing so fast that you cannot eat enough to keep from getting hungry. See if you notice that your mood swings are in some way connected to your eating certain foods or not eating at all. See if your "laziness" in the morning is a function of what you ate before bedtime. See if skin trouble comes and goes with chocolate, sugar, or whatever is your favorite. Notice what foods give you gas. How long are you straining to have bowel movement? Notice how tight your rings get after eating salty foods; your brain could be swelling up inside your skull and giving you that terrible headache.

This is called reading the body. Most of us take until the age of 40 years or so to get that "Aha!" insight into how the body works and what things are doing what to our bodies. If we continue to be rude to our bodies by eating nutrient-impoverished food, not exercising, not getting enough rest, doing too much, and drinking alcohol or taking drugs, Mother Nature will strike back and dump some painful disease on us.

The rapid growing years of puberty and adolescence demand huge numbers of calories. But in order for the body to use these calories, B complex, calcium, magnesium, and about 40 other nutrients are required almost every day. It is no time to be eating nutrient-poor foods. For instance, zinc is fairly abundant in whole grains, seafood, liver, peas, carrots, and nuts, and less so in other foods; it is usually absent in food that has been processed.

Zinc is necessary as an enzyme activator for about 50 or more functions of the body. A zinc deficiency has been found to be linked to the following conditions: acne, poor growth, delayed or absent sexual organ development, poor wound healing, distorted sense of taste and smell, hyperactivity, epilepsy, body and breath odor, etc. Dr. Carl Pfeiffer[1] summarizes the importance of zinc during periods of rapid growth and sexual maturation: "Zinc is required for normal pubertal development of the male, and deficiency may cause a growth lag." For the teenage girl, "at a time when zinc is lowest and copper is high, premenstrual tension occurs."

I have been seeing a number of adolescents and adults who felt they were eating three good meals a day and still showed evidence of a deficiency in one or several of the 40 or so nutrients that our bodies need. The topsoil from which our foods draw their nourishment is disappearing and becoming depleted of the trace minerals that our enzyme systems need. In addition, the enzymes present in the lining cells of our intestinal tract require these minerals and vitamins so they can digest and absorb the foods that we send down to them. Nutrient-poor, processed food from a deficient soil will have an effect sooner or later. Many people find themselves gaining weight because they are eating more calorie-dense foods in an effort to get all the trace minerals their body cries out for.

Children who eat dirt are looking for iron and zinc. People who love to chew ice are often anemic. Check it out. Adults over 40 find they cannot eat the large slices of meat that they did as youths; they do not have the same amount of stomach acid and

---

[1] *Mental and Elemental Nutrients* (New Canaan, Conn: Keats Publishing, 1975.)

the hunk of protein and gristle sits there giving them the bloat. Most over-50-year-old adults cannot eat the same amount of food that they did when growing; their metabolism has slowed. I do some aerobic exercise every other day but still have to cut down on the calories. My margin of metabolic safety is very narrow.

Adolescents can often eat just about anything because all their juices are flowing abundantly and they are burning up the calories and building the muscles and organs. But after 15 to 17 years of age the growth spurt is slowing down and an effort should be made to cut down the intake accordingly. The fats, the sugars, and the salt are the chief antinutrients. Remember, it requires B vitamins and a few of the minerals to make the digestive enzymes work efficiently. If you have eaten empty calories for a while, your gut may not be the efficient machine you thought it was. You may have friends who seem to be able to eat everything and anything without trouble, but you might be amazed to find out as I have how revoltingly malodorous and huge their bowel movements are. They are having some trouble with absorption and that could be due to the tired intestinal enzymes that have not gotten the proper amount of B vitamins and minerals to do the job. Or they are eating some food to which they are allergic, and it just sits down there in the hollow tunnels of the gut—the victim of putrefying bacteria. Sometimes the person's breath gives this away.

Crash diets that emphasize but one food group or limit the foods to just protein (or those protein drinks) or just fruit are especially dangerous during these periods of rapid growth. Many of us are on the edge of vitamin and mineral deficiency and a sickness or a poor diet may push us into an obvious, embarrassing disaster. If we all were working on the farm and burning 6,000 calories a day, and eating a variety of good foods, we would probably be getting all the vitamins and minerals that we need for these enzyme systems. But because we ride, and sit, and stare into space a lot, we may gain if we eat more than 2,000 to 2,500 calories a day. It has been estimated that if one cuts one's calorie consumption below 1,800 calories a day in an effort to lose weight, it is virtually impossible to get all the needed vitamins and minerals, even if one eats the best that nature can provide. We probably all should take a supplement, and some of us need bigger doses of some of the supplements.

Let me illustrate what I used to do for adolescents in my *early* days of practice:

Many of my patients, like Laura, had bodies built like blocks: square and big and noticeable. Laura tried to reduce by only drinking water for four days, but she got so tired and depressed she had to quit. When she was 14 her mother brought (dragged and pushed) her in to have me, the expert, straighten (thin) her out. Her mother was a powerful Katrinka (like the Valkyrie) type herself. (Their ancestry happened to be middle European, but the body type is almost universal.) The examination was okay, but her weight was 160 pounds and her height was only 5 feet 2 inches, not quite what is considered within the normal limits of height-weight ratios. I, of course, wanted to impress them with the medical knowledge I had gained in medical school.

"What is breakfast?" I asked.

"One egg, one piece of unbuttered toast, and a glass of orange juice."

No more than 150 to 200 calories, I figured.

"How about lunch?"

"One salad, no dressing, and two tablespoons of cottage cheese."

"Okay," I stalled. This is going to be tough. Let's see, about 100 calories there. "Dinner?"

"Three ounces of meat or fish, some steamed veggies, one small baked potato—no dressing or butter—tea, and a cup of yogurt and fruit for dessert."

Four hundred calories at the most. She must be cheating. Now I've got it.

"What about snacks before bedtime?"

"Maybe an apple or ten almonds."

This girl must be manufacturing calories in her intestines somehow. I tried another tact, exercise.

"Do you have gym at school?"

"Oh, yes, it's required. We swim or jog around the track or do aerobic exercises for fifteen minutes three times a week."

Gulp. This is getting serious. I'm scraping the bottom of my knowledge barrel of what to do. I'm a pediatrician, an expert. I remember the nutrition axiom: Eat three meals a day and something from the four food groups, and eat a little less of everything. The oracle speaks.

Well, that's how it was in the good old days. The doctor knew the answer and if it didn't work, it meant that the *patient* was not cooperating. We weren't very helpful to people like Laura some years ago.

Now let's see what we could do for an overweight adolescent today.

I start by observing body type: a heavy young person is most likely to be an endomorph. He or she will have thickish lips and short, tapering fingers. These people are likely to have a long intestinal tract that increases absorption of food. Long thin body types are usually ectomorphs who rarely get fat, and the vigorous, muscular, broad mesomorphs usually don't begin to get fat until they stop exercising, usually after they're thirty or so years old.

Next I would ask my overweight patient the following questions:

1. Is there obesity in the family?

    If both parents are obese, 80 percent of the children will have a struggle with their weight all their lives.

2. Were you heavy from age 6 to 11? Only 10 percent of fat-looking babies grow up to be heavy adults. If, however, a child was overweight from age 6 to age 11, he or she will have to fight the weight battle all his or her life.

3. Are your hands and feet cold to the touch? Do you wear socks to bed? Do you put a sweater on in the summer when others are comfortable in blouse or shirt sleeves? Are you sluggish and have trouble getting out of bed even after 10 hours sleep? Are you constipated even when off the dairy products?

    If you answer yes to most of these, you are probably hypothyroid despite a normal blood test. We suggest that you get a prescription for thyroid medication from your doctor. You may only need the medication for a few months.

4. Is there some food that you eat every day because you love it?

    It may be that you are allergic to that food, nutritious though it may be, and it is causing your blood sugar to fall. This sugar is stored as fat; a weight problem may develop. The most common allergy-causers are the dairy products, then corn, soy, wheat, eggs, shellfish, and nuts.

5. Are you noticing stress?

    Everyone has some stress or we would not be reacting to or even noticing our environment. A girl sitting in my cold examining room in her underwear talking to a fully clothed adult male would be experiencing some kind of stress.

Today, I often encounter the following response to asking "Laura" if she's aware of stress in her life:

"I don't know," she says, and glances at her mother.

Her mother answers for her: "She sometimes spends hours in her room. Occasionally a classmate calls. I try to offer support, but she tells me I don't understand. Her father died of a heart attack four years ago. I do understand; I was like that when I was her age."

I figure I'm going to have to be the extended family here. I don't know what to do medically except to get a thyroid blood test, but I can at least offer an outlet, a friendly hand, a psychic prop. I'd hate to have a patient of mine get dangerously depressed because life seemed to be a boring, endless drag.

I decide it would be better to talk to the daughter alone. (I have found over the years that the real message is expressed in eye contact, not by words. I can let her know that I think she is important and help her communicate. I can do that because my mother thought I was okay despite mood swings, bed-wetting, and immature behavior.)

"Get dressed, Laura; I want to talk to you." Babies are screaming in the waiting room, but I read somewhere that children and adolescents will sometimes believe the doctor before they will believe their parents or their teachers. I try to do it right.

So now it is just Laura and I. "Well, tell me, Laura, do you laugh and smile more than you cry and frown?" This is sometimes a good way to start a counseling session.

"I dunno," she murmurs.

"Do you have a friend or two to talk to?"

"I guess," is her slow response.

"Are you worried about your body, your size, your health, your grades, your future, your friends, your whatever?" I tick them off.

"Sort of," she shrugs.

"Look, if you have trouble talking about it, let me give you my phone number so that you can call me when you have some questions formulated. This is just between you and me; I am your doctor and I want to be helpful, but because I am an adult, you may think I am not to be trusted. We'll check your thyroid, but at the same time take your morning temperature by mouth or armpit before you get out of bed. It should be 98°, or at least no lower than 97.6°. I'll call you next week and see what you find and I'll tell you about the blood test." I'm groping, but I'm leaving the door open.

I have Laura sit in the waiting room while I am talking to her mother. "She seems subdued." I am searching. "Does she talk to you?"

"Only if she wants something. I have to work to hold things together and I'm bushed when I get home. Who holds me together? She's usually in her room and I know that she's lonely and bitter about her body size. She's built like me when I was her age."

I tell Laura's mother to encourage Laura to call me at the first sign of indifference, depression, boredom, loneliness, or other inappropriate behavior. I explain the deficiences in their diet, and that both of them would be better off with the six-meals-a-day, nibbling approach to eating. No milk, cut back on the beef, get sugar out of the house, and both of them are to snack on vegetables, as little cooked as possible, fruit, seeds, nuts, whole grain cereals and breads, and some fish and chicken. A big capsule of the B complex, a tablet with 1,000 mg of vitamin C, and 1,000 mg of calcium and 1,000 mg of magnesium are urged on both of them every day.

I call in one week and again in 4 weeks. Mother and daughter are pleasantly surprised to find that they are more cheerful, they get out of bed more easily in the morning, they have less gas, they don't use so many tissues, and they both have lost a little weight (5 pounds for each), and, wonder of wonders, Laura is calling her friends and laughs a lot. The temperature in the morning is about 97.4° to 97.6° for Laura; because she feels better I am going to wait before prescribing the thyroid medication. But Mom is down to 97°, so I call in a prescription for thyroid (Armour's desiccated, 1 grain daily); she feels great in about 3 weeks. I may even suggest a few B-complex shots to get their metabolisms going after years of eating impoverished foods.

I feel sorry that I had nothing to offer to the heavy adolescent in the early days of my practice—except guilt. Now we can offer hope to the Lauras of the world.

I have placed these examples of office visits in this chapter so the reader can get an idea of the general attitude and interest of the doctor that is so necessary in dealing with the teenager who is on the edge of paranoia and depression. If your doctor is not fulfilling his role of the kindly supportive educator, search for another, or find a psychologist or a minister or priest who would at least be empathic.

TO THE TEENAGER: To a certain extent you are stuck with your genes, but you can do the best to make your body work optimally inside that configuration. What you see in the mirror is what you get. What is thin? What is normal? Doctors have tables of optimum height and weight recommendations. We know if you exceed the weight for your height, you are at risk for certain degenerative diseases. High blood pressure, diabetes, varicosities, and cancer of the colon, breast, and uterus are more common in heavier people.

What you may perceive in yourself as fat may really be only your bones and muscles and some fat that is forming around you. You feel klutzy because you are not used to the outer limits of your body. You don't know where you end. You hit your hips against the door frame and snag your clothes. Your nerves do not grow as fast as your bones and muscles. It is new and uncomfortable.

In Covert Bailey's *Fit or Fat* (Boston: Houghton Mifflin Company, 1978) he describes the normal adult female as having about 22 to 23 percent of her body weight as fat. The male should be at about 15 percent fat. There are special ways to measure this but probably the easiest test that you can do at home is to lie flat on the floor and put a yardstick on your chest and your pubic bone (that first bone about 6 inches below your navel). If the yardstick can touch your chest and your pubic bone without touching your abdomen, then you are probably not overweight. If you can pinch up the skin on the back of your arm and it is no thicker than about one inch, you are probably not overly fat.

We older adults want you young people to be healthy and take care of us in our old age, but we mainly want you to have a good self-image. We don't want you to be thin and scrawny; it is unhealthy. We don't want you to be fat and depressed either. We are sorry if we gave you some bad genes that make weight control difficult. We love you; we are all in this together. With a little faith and a good diet, we all will survive and even laugh more than we cry.

CHAPTER 2

Reading Your Own Body (Or, Figuring Out Your Physiology)

TO THE TEENAGER: Most parents dread to see their children approaching the teen years. It may be because they remember their own personal miseries and are reluctant to see their loved ones traveling through a rough time. They well remember the fights they had with their own parents over their drive for freedom and some autonomy. They remember how everything and everyone seemed to be against them. Even nature seemed to be plotting against them at that age and endowed them with acne, stringy hair, or bad breath. Fatigue and crabbiness for no reason seemed to be almost daily events, and their parents and counselors told them it was hormones, or just a stage, but no explanation made them feel any better.

You may have noticed that some of your friends are sailing through these years with a minimum of sickness, anxiety, pain, depression, and noncompliance, which suggests that feeling good may be normal, albeit not average. Many of the conditions you teenagers have are controllable, and diet has much to do with them. It is important for you to consider what you are eating now, what you ate as a little child, and what your mother ate during her pregnancy with you.

Once you begin to learn a little bit about nutrition you will see that the way you feel and look is not entirely up to fate. If the body looks and feels good, that is its way of saying you are treating it well. If you could look or feel better, chances are there are changes you could make, and this is the body's way of telling you. Listen!

Childhood Antecedents

Much of the way we act toward our peer group and parents and the way we feel about ourselves as adolescents and adults is determined by the messages we got from our parents when we were infants and children. The test of time has indicated that the feelings of acceptance or rejection instilled in us in those early years become internalized and have long-term effects on the way we care about ourselves throughout our whole lives. If your mother was depressed for one reason or another or thought you were the wrong sex or you had an irritating cry, you might have gotten the impression that you were unacceptable, and even on that first day of life, you might have asked, "Why was I born?"

You may have been whiny because you had a bad head-ache, but your mother probably tried to cuddle and love you despite her postpartum miseries. She may have refused most of the painkiller drugs during delivery because she wanted you to be bright and alert. Even so, your brightness and alertness might have turned to colic and sleep reversal and general fussiness. So she may have tried to feed you every hour night and day; that didn't work. She may have tried to let you scream it out at night under the assumption that you just had "a bad habit." You might have gotten hot and sweaty and even broken a few capillaries on your face from the straining. Your parents felt guilty. Your sleep-wakefulness cycles didn't jibe with the rhythm of the house.

Some of this turmoil might have been prevented if your mother had eaten differently during pregnancy. Pregnant women must eat a variety of nutrient-dense foods every day. Protein, complex carbohydrates, some fats, and extra vitamins and minerals will more likely produce a healthy, allergy-free baby. Primitive people knew this; it was part of their cultural heritage. The ancients ate nuts, seeds, fruit, vegetables, wild game, fish, fowl, and, more recently, whole grains. They had no junk foods nor did they eat impoverished, nutritionally empty foods. Mountain people went to the seashore to gather fish and iodine-containing foods for their pregnant women. Many used dolomite (calcium and magnesium carbonate) to help grind the grain. The tribe gave emotional support to the pregnant women; they knew if the woman had a healthy body and a stress-free nine months, she would more likely have a healthy, robust child, free of infections.

Touchy, sensitive, goosey, wakeful babies are frequently the victims of inadequate storage of calcium and magnesium (zinc and manganese, also) before birth. I wonder how many infants might get battered because they cannot stop crying because they simply do not feel good. And their misery can be traced to an inadequate or inappropriate diet during pregnancy. If the mother consumed a great deal of milk during pregnancy, the large intake may have set her baby up for a milk allergy. (I'll discuss alternative sources of calcium for pregnant mothers later in this chapter.) Ingestion of foods to which one is sensitive will distort and damage the intestinal lining cells necessary to digest and absorb those ingredients in that allergenic food. The food sits there, the victim of intestinal bacterial action. Result: fermentation of carbohydrates, rancidification of fats, and putrefaction of protein: smelly gas, bad breath.

I feel guilty now when I see the parents of some of my ex-patients. They say; "You were my child's doctor!"

"Whoops," I gulp. "Is he all right?"

"Oh, sure," they reassure me. "He seems okay."

I breathe a sigh of relief. A doctor did not always know what was going on thirty years ago when a mother reported that her child was irritable, colicky, wakeful. All we knew to do then was to stone the poor thing with a sedative. If they had come in with an obvious ear infection, a broken bone, or even kala-azar, we could have been helpful, because those are the diseases we were trained to diagnose and to treat.

Now I know that nutrition is one of the hidden factors. To some extent this simplifies matters. There is less need to search about, as we used to, for some esoteric psychiatric screw-up that might have produced the child's noncompliant behavior.

Sometimes babies, just like their parents, develop colic or other intestinal disorders due to stress. Being a baby isn't as easy as it looks. Life in the womb was much more carefree; there were so many fewer adult vibrations. If the lining of the baby's intestinal tract has been damaged due to stress, a malnourished pregnancy, or a milk allergy, the ability to absorb the nutriments from cow's milk (and even from the cow's milk in the breast-fed baby whose mother drinks it while nursing) is compromised. In those first few months the growth rate is at its peak, and poor absorption of calcium, magnesium, zinc, and manganese will lead to chronic irritability, sleeplessness, bedrocking, thumb-sucking, spitting up, occasional vomiting, and stiff-arming the parents.

The parents try to soothe their infant but the child pushes himself away as if they are too close. The parents hold their baby because he is crying; but the baby may associate his distress with being held. Will that child learn, somehow, that his parents caused the crying? (See how nutrition can appear to be a psychiatric tilt? A calcium and magnesium deficiency can sometimes cause the world to appear close and threatening.)

In the twenties and early thirties the best medical advice was to feed children every four hours during the day so they would develop "good habits." But a lot of those babies had not read the books, so they went merrily on upsetting their parents' best plans. Resentments might have crept in (on both sides). But the good Lord made babies so cute that one cannot begrudge them a little crying time. Not all parents, however, feel secure enough emotionally, physically, and financially to be the all-caring, all-loving, all-accepting warm parents that they are told they *should* be.

The point is that many infants, because of a nutritional problem, simply do not feel good. Their moodiness and irritability may sabotage the development of their own self-image. It's a vicious cycle. If they are touchy and uncuddlable, parents tend to leave them alone. If they and their mothers had had the optimum amounts of the vitamins and minerals, they might have felt so good and might have shown such pleasure when snuggled that their overjoyed parents would have snuggled and loved them even more. What a great way to glide through a rapid growing period: eating, sleeping, and getting cuddled.

You adolescents with any sort of health problem, physical or mental, should make some effort—before your parents forget—

to find out more about those early months. Much of what happens in your teen years could be explained by information about your infancy. It is possible that the way you feel now as an adolescent may have some antecedents in your infancy or childhood. People are not congenitally crabby; something makes that happen.

One possible explanation for a number of the health and mood difficulties of the adolescent may be a milk allergy. Cow's milk sensitivity usually shows up in the infant as colic. If your mother says that you had colic, but you were being nursed, it still could be from the cow as she may have been eating cheese, yogurt, or ice cream, or drinking milk, during the time that she was nursing you.

Fermented milk products, like yogurt and buttermilk, seem to be less irritating than milk, and these are excellent sources of calcium and protein. Goat's milk is an even better source than cow's milk. But if you want to stay away from dairy products altogether, there are plenty of other foods that are high in calcium. One cup of dried figs (careful! could be a purge for some) has about the same amount of calcium as an equal volume of milk. Leafy greens, like chard, mustard greens, collard, and kale are extremely good sources. Black beans and chick peas, broccoli and corn tortillas are good sources of calcium.

If you had a number of ear infections as an infant or child, or you had croup or asthma or bronchitis, they were probably triggered by a milk allergy. The body tries to get the owner to pay attention. If the colicky baby's caretakers do not change the milk because they do not believe that a milk allergy causes colic, then the body moves the mischief to another organ system; asthma might be the next disturbing symptom to show up. Bed-wetting may be the next signal that the allergy is still around. Some will start to have nosebleeds or migraines when the bed-wetting stops. Many adolescents and adults constantly clear their throats or drive everyone up the wall with an irritating, dry cough that goes on night and day. All due to allergies. Look to your own body for some clues that mean nutrient deficiencies or food allergies that correlate with problems your folks will tell you occurred when you were an infant.

If you had a milk allergy and thought you outgrew it, it may now reappear because of your rapid growth in adolescence. Are you drinking more? Sometimes it's tough to get off a food you love. But a craving often suggests that you are allergic and addicted to that food. It takes three weeks of no milk, cheese, ice cream—no diary products whatsoever—to get rid of the symptoms. Milk is the number one food allergy in our country; only the dairy council thinks you should drink it every day. But remember to get an alternative source of calcium once you're off dairy products.

You may notice that if you stay away from corn your acne is better. Food allergies can cause anything. The worst part of all this is that the food that is causing your distress, stomach aches, diarrhea, constipation, fatigue, napping in class, frequent colds, wheeze, and skin rashes, depression or surliness, is usually the food that you love the most and try to eat every day.

I recall a patient of mine, a 10-year-old farm boy who loved milk and drank about a gallon a day (that's four quarts). He was a little rotund, but not really out of line. His main complaint was daily headaches. We figured, as you must have guessed, that it was the milk. We made him stop it, and after two to three weeks of milk abstinence, his headaches were gone. He had never felt so good in his life. After this little bit of successful detective work, the parents had to shell out good money to feed the boy; the milk had been free, the groceries were not. "Okay, we've proved that milk causes headaches, so go back to it. The headaches weren't *that* bad, were they?" they asked him.

"I love the way I feel now. I'll never touch the stuff again." The dark circles disappeared from his lower lids, he had more energy, and his breath didn't smell dead anymore.

Try to analyze your own symptoms. What troubles do you have that you would like to get rid of? What parts of your body are you ashamed of? What mental or physical functions do you think could be improved upon? There are some things that you may have to put up with because they are genetic or run in the family. But nutrition can assuage the impact of genetic traits; it is not as hopeless as you thought.

Family Tendencies

I have spent a great deal of my career as a physician trying to figure out if a child's or adolescent's problems are due to inherited or genetic factors, or to psychiatric problems, or if they could be due to nutritional deficiencies. Most, I would judge, are a combination.

My father was a headache person; he died of high blood pressure and a stroke. I have headaches when stress and a poor diet hit me simultaneously. I don't want to suffer a stroke. Dad ate salt, he smoked, drank rum and cola, and had me as a son. Stress. But a good diet can allow one to ignore the stresses of one's life.

Low Blood Sugar (Hypoglycemia)

If your family has a high incidence of diabetes, obesity, or alcoholism, and you fall on the floor after you have eaten a candy bar, you probably have the family curse—hypoglycemia. It's no big deal, but you need to be nibbling six times a day on vegetables, fruits, nuts, seeds, whole grains, and bits of fish and fowl—and cutting out the candy bars. Here is a short list of the symptoms that may be associated with low blood sugar: nervousness, irritability, exhaustion, dizziness, tremor, cold sweats, depression, drowsiness, headaches, forgetfulness, heart palpitations, confusion, and crying spells. Are you in there somewhere? Do you have mood swings? Are you a Jekyll-and-Hyde type of person?

Most of the above symptoms can be eliminated or reduced in severity by eating good foods at frequent intervals. Their ingestion usually provides optimum energy and cheerfulness at a fairly constant level.

Obesity

Obesity can run in families. Look at your parents. If they are portly and their lives seem to center about the dinner table, you may be genetically trapped. If you were overweight from age 6 to 12, you are probably overweight now, and the genetic influences may have already shown up, but it is not the end of the world. Nutritional science has found some answers for you, but you have to accept the fact that you are different from your friends who are long and thin and seem to be able to eat anything. You have a different body build and you cannot change that.

Look at your parents again, and, if possible, take a close look at your grandparents. What do the ones who most resemble you have as their chronic problem? Can they eat anything and stay cheerful, energetic, and maintain a normal weight? Or are they glum, tired, and chubby?

Alcoholism

If you resemble the family member who needs two drinks every day or there seems to be a lot of drinking amongst your relatives, you don't have to be doomed to be an alcoholic.

Genetic factors can almost force children into the sauce. Adolescents are less likely to abuse alcohol if their parents are dry, and, as a corollary, if relatives drink, youngsters are more likely to accept drinking as a lifestyle. An adolescent is almost doomed if, coupled with the family tendencies he or she has peer pressure, wants to assert a degree of independence, and wants to calm sexual anxieties and reduce depression ("Survey: Alcoholism and the Family," *Human Sexuality*, vol. 18, Sept. 1984, pp. 177–187).

In those with the family trait, one drink is too many and a thousand are not enough. If a poor self-esteem has weakened the psychic underpinnings, a little stress (or the perception that things are stressful) can push anyone into the alcohol trap. It is a condoned remedy—an easy but potentially fatal out!

If you have alcoholics in your family and you have had a bad experience with the stuff, we know that low blood sugar is a big factor and the craving for another drink is the response to this empty feeling. The ingestion of small amounts of nutrient-dense food will help to maintain the blood sugar at a level high enough to prevent the desire for booze to be so compelling.

Alcoholics lose all the B vitamins, but especially thiamine (B_1). A deficiency of this frequently leads to impulsive behavior. Magnesium also runs out of the body when alcohol is ingested; magnesium deficiency leads to depression, anxiety, and a low threshold for noise. These feelings and perceptions can make one need a drink; a vicious cycle.

Rats fed the American diet of white flour, sugar, beef, and fat tended to drink alcohol although water was also provided in their cages. Rats fed good laboratory chow disregarded the alcohol and drank the water. Eating nutrient-poor foods at infrequent intervals may push a genetically susceptible but latent alcoholic into the manifest disease.

Glutamine, 1,000–3,000 mg a day, can help maintain abstinence. Gamma linolenic acid helps. Exposure to chemical, solvent, gasoline, and formaldehyde fumes can set up the compulsion for an alcoholic drink.

Allergies

If your family all seem to be well and happy, but you are a sniveling, sickly, drippy-nosed, pale, coughing, wheezing, miserable mess, it may mean that your mother or you had some stress along the way—often at the time of birth. Maybe the cord was around your neck. Maybe you were a breech delivery. Some physical, emotional, climatic trauma sufficient to deplete your adrenal glands is all it takes to give a person a lifetime of allergies. And the stress of the symptoms of the allergy is enough to further the adrenal gland exhaustion which, of course, would continue the allergy.

Find out about the allergies in your family. The usual sneezing and wheezing suggest an inhalation allergy and may be quieted by dumping the cat, shutting off the hot air register, or exchanging the feather pillow. But if you have done the environmental control and your tissues are still swollen and itchy, you might consider helping your adrenal glands with a nutritional approach. You might be amazed at what you can do for yourself with vitamin C, pantothenic acid, some vitamin A, and no sugar.

Food allergies are hard to diagnose, but frequent illnesses usually indicate immune-system weaknesses which are based on food sensitivities. The most common food allergy is to milk. It takes three weeks to get all the dairy products out of the system. If the dairy is your enemy, you would begin to notice a clear head and open respiratory passages in that time. Many find that fatigue lifts, cheeks become pink, dark circles under the eyes disappear, and the overweight tendency becomes controllable. Remember, if you ingest foods to which you are allergic, your blood sugar will bounce up and down, leading to anxiety, hunger, depression, fatigue, irritability, and weight gain. The foods you love the most are usually the ones to which you are sensitive. It is called the allergic-addictive syndrome.

Food sensitivities are infrequently diagnosed by skin tests. Blood tests (RAST, cytotoxic) are reasonably reliable, but many people can figure out their own allergies by reading the body. Anything can do anything. The most common symptom I note in food-sensitive people is a Jekyll-and-Hyde tendency. Ups and downs. Mood swings for no good reason.

If you have gone through the miseries of skin testing and are getting the de-sensitizing shots and little is happening to control your allergies, you and your parents might consider the modern intradermal quantitative skin tests which provide the information for the neutralizing doses of the offending allergens that you can safely take at home. But short of that there are some diet and nutritional things that you can do to assuage that cough, sneeze, sniff, itch, and wheeze.

I have seen good results when I take my allergy-prone patients off dairy products, eggs, wheat, soy, and corn. Because these foods so often cause allergies they become a burden to the control system of the body; with them not overtaxing the homeostasis of the body, the symptoms due to house dust or grass pollens may disappear.

Vitamin C (2,000 to 10,000 mg, depending on bowel action), calcium, magnesium (1,000 mg of each, best near bedtime), vitamin B_6 (50 to 200 mg a day, until dream recall is good), pantothenic acid (500 to 1,000 mg a day), vitamin A (20,000 units a day for a month and then every other day), zinc (30 to 60 mg a day for a month) and histidine can be helpful in building your adrenals back into functioning at their optimum level. Rotating the diet is always a good idea, whether you are allergic or not. Vary the diet. Try to reduce the consumption of any food to once every four days. This allows the body to rest and restore itself. Eating the same foods every day tends to produce sensitivities to those foods. The body becomes addicted and that is a stress. If you have allergies, try to eliminate the food you love the most or are eating daily. Substitute rye crackers for bread; rice cereal for wheat. Increase your intake of leafy green vegetables. Get your protein from beans instead of cheeseburgers for a while. If you ate a banana today for your fruit, try a melon tomorrow, an apple the next day, then an orange, and then repeat the banana. Don't deprive yourself, but try to rotate and substitute.

Adolescent Problems: A Nutritional Approach

One nice thing about being a human being is that one has a brain to help solve problems. If you feel a pain when you walk, you would take your shoe off and look for a piece of gravel that may have found its way in. If you get sick a lot, your immune system is faulty and you would benefit from taking a course of increased vitamin C, which helps the body make interferon, a natural intracellular, antiviral substance.

If you have an infection, you might want to treat it, but at the same time it seems logical to want to know why you got sick in the first place. Ask yourself, "Why?" Then ask the doctor. It has been established that zinc helps an enzyme in the skin that lays down protein; if you are low in zinc, you might have skin trouble.

If you have cavities in your teeth, it is average, but it is not normal. Assume that a tilt has occurred in the way your body is functioning, and make an effort to correct it.

What to Do If You Have Trouble with Your Memory, or If You Are Behind In Your Schoolwork and Everyone Says You Are Smart Enough to Do the Work

The brain is run by enzymes; these are chemical compounds that have the ability to manufacture other chemicals that are excreted at the ends of the nerves and stimulate other nerves which retrieve memory, move muscles, secrete hormones, and do the work of the body. These enzymes must have energy to do their work, a constant supply of energy. The growing brain needs about twice the amount that an adult brain needs. This energy comes from food, of course, but the energy is best supplied over a long period of time. Quick energy from sugar or a candy bar or a soft drink raises the blood sugar so rapidly that the pancreas excretes its hormone, insulin, which rapidly drives the sugar into storage in the muscles and the liver—but starves the brain. The victim goes to sleep or acts stupid or drugged, or craves a sugar fix.

Foods we eat should provide enough energy for at least two to four hours. Because the sugar in fruit or the starch in vegetables is locked up inside the food, it takes a while for the energy to get out of the food, be broken down into simple sugars, absorbed into the circulation, and spread to the body and brain cells. The best example is the apple. When a person eats an apple, the sugar level in his or her blood slowly rises and falls over a period of three to five hours. Applesauce, on the other hand, allows the sugar to get into the bloodstream in less than an hour, and the blood sugar rises higher than after the apple is eaten. The fall is also faster, and ends at a lower level. When apple juice is drunk, the blood sugar shoots up in just 20 to 30 minutes; the pancreas does not like this, so it squirts out insulin and the blood sugar drops very rapidly; moreover, the level may drop exceedingly low and produce symptoms of hyperactivity, lethargy, migraine, hives, and some oddball mental symptoms, chief of which is depression. The fiber, pectins, and roughage in the whole apple prevent the rapid uptake of the sugar; the energy is provided over a longer period of time.

There is a definite connection between the ingestion of sugary foods and criminality.[2] Apparently when the blood sugar falls because of this overproduction of insulin, the part of the brain called the conscience is no longer operating well enough for some of us to avoid antisocial behavior.

The trick, then, is to do some detective work and see if your ability to function mentally is at all related to the food you are eating. Your ability to think and learn is dependent on the flow of energy through the brain; that's sugar and water and oxygen. But the sources must be fairly constant. If you get tired, or depressed, or surly for no good reason, think quickly about the last meal you had; some food in that meal is allowing your blood sugar to drop. Anything can do anything.

Drowsiness During the Day

The worst time most students have is that 1:00 P.M. class right after lunch. The teacher is droning on about the "sweep of history," and you would just as soon be home taking a nap. Or you find yourself napping right in the classroom. When this happened to me I blamed the boring teacher, but now that I

[2] Barbara Reed, *Food, Teens and Behavior* (Manitowoc, Wis.: Natural Press, 1983.)

know a few things I find that it was the jelly sandwiches on white bread that put me away. They should have been peanut butter on whole grain bread.

Because most diets are nutritionally unsound, they can put people into a state of semistarvation and cause the same sleepy or manic states that sugary foods cause (after all, animals attack when they are hungry). When you diet, if you are not completely drained and sunken-eyed, you are in a bad mood. There is nothing in your blood to perk you up. Nobody ever enjoys a diet; you sit there while the history teacher drones on, thinking about how hungry you are and about all the things you'd like to eat but can't.

The answer here is, don't diet. If you eat the right foods and get exercise, you won't need to, especially since you now know that the body you have is the one you inherited, and, given a proper diet and plenty of activity, it's the one you're going to live with. If this idea fills you with despair, remember also that during the teenage years your body is in a state of flux, the flesh is moving around to the places where it will be useful later, but it may not have settled yet. And don't forget, hardly anybody really looks like the models on the cover of *Vogue*.

Give it a whirl. Try some of the snacks that Martha Rose has provided here in the book and see if you handle the postlunch slump a little better. You may still have a boring teacher, but you won't be embarrassed by falling asleep. You can stay awake and write letters to friends, or draw pictures while pretending that you are taking notes.

Fatigue After Eight Hours of Sleep

One of the quickest ways to find out if some of your mental symptoms are due to a food allergy or to hypoglycemia from the ingestion of sugary nothings is to eat some meat, almonds, peanuts, or some such long-acting energy source at bedtime. Then see if you can get out of bed more easily and more cheerfully in the morning after but seven or eight hours of restful sleep. You should know your name, what day of the week it is, and where you put your socks the night before. Try it and let me know.

Bad Dreams

You might find that your bad dreams are related to what you eat from suppertime on. If you eat a sugary dessert or snack while watching a late movie, or you eat something to which you are allergic, your blood sugar may fall so fast through the night that your body assumes some threat is imminent and pumps out adrenalin to get ready for flight or fight. But there is no monster out there. The adrenalin makes a normal dream about school or *Star Wars* a real nightmare. You may awaken with dilated pupils and rapid heartbeat, drenched in sweat. It is not psychogenic; it is biochemical.

Your feeling of anxiety or impending doom may be this same adrenalin release two to four hours after a doughnut, a candy bar, or a bowl of Sugar Frosted Flakes. Many students hate school because of these frightening anxiety attacks. You don't need counseling; you need a better breakfast. School can be a boring drag even without a biochemical tilt mucking up one's perception.

Depression for No Good Reason

Almost every week the newspapers report the high suicide rate among the teenage population. Next to accidents, it is the most common cause of death in your age group. And for every one death by suicide there are about 10 adolescents who have tried pills, cutting arteries, or hanging themselves, and survived. It is a terrible waste, and all parents worry that their child will do such a foolish thing.

I can remember getting very depressed at odd times when I was growing up—when there was no particular reason for feeling so down. Some days it was that a longtime friend was talking animatedly to another classmate. "He never talked that way to me! He doesn't like me any more. What's the point of going on?" But somehow I did.

Emotional memories are stored by categories: laughter, scary things, disgusting things, beautiful things, and depressing things. Once someone or something slides a person into one of the categories, the person seems to "notice" other similar groupings. The teenager has mood swings anyway, and because he or she takes things so seriously and intensely, an unintentional slight may seem to signify the termination of a friendship for all time. Now he is nudged into the "hurt" mode, and the teenager finds it an easy slide into the "depressed" mode, where all the other depressing events in his life hang like pictures on a wall in a broad, flattened apartment in his brain. Each one makes him, the owner of these memories, feel so worthless and unimportant that the poor dejected youth feels he might as well do himself in.

Nutritional therapists believe that the ingestion of sugary foods or foods to which a person is allergic will cause depression as deep as that caused by the loss of a loved one. If you become saddened for no really valid reason, think of what you have been eating, especially something that you like. Some have found that taking extra vitamin B_3 will improve their outlook. Nutritional research has discovered that a magnesium deficiency can produce a profound depression. Magnesium deficiency is common in our country, and drug-takers and alcoholics will lose the mineral rapidly. It is found in green vegetables and most seeds and nuts.

The B-complex vitamins may be the single most important factor for the health of the nerves, and they are also active in supplying the factors for the enzymes that turn food into energy.

I have found it necessary to give some of my patients shots of the B complex with special emphasis on folic acid and B_{12} before they responded to psychotherapy and a good diet.

In my experience the greatest factor in teenage suicide is Pyroluria—a stress-induced deficiency in both zinc and vitamin B_6. The onset of this disorder is around ages 15 to 17. With a deficiency in both B_6 and zinc, the teenager is confused, depressed, and sleepless. If he mentions this to his peers or parents, he may be taunted or scolded or suspected of abusing alcohol or drugs. If he sees a therapist, too much emphasis may be placed on a lack of friends or "too much" social interaction. The real cause is a family tendency to Pyroluria, the mineral needs of body growth, the eating of junk foods which contain no minerals, and an overall stressful time of life. The stress can come from the first sex encounter, the pressure of school work or numerous other teenage problems which, at the time, seem insoluble.

Pyroluria is caused by the excretion of a definite chemical—

Kryptopyrrole. Fully 20% of normal people excrete Kryptopyrrole which takes with it zinc, vitamin B_6, and perhaps manganese. A concerted effort must be made to devise a good diet with adequate amounts of these nutrients, since they're not found in the processed foods of the most common American diet. A supplement of 15 mg of zinc, 10 mg of manganese and 100 mg, or more, of vitamin B_6 will usually correct all the symptoms of Pyrroluria within one week's time.

A second biological cause of suicide is the presence of too much histamine in the body (the histadelic person). Histamine is liberated in the allergic reaction and causes excess secretions throughout the body. We do know that allergies run in families. Sometimes, these family members with allergies have more than the usual amount of energy and impulsiveness and are often self starters. But these active people may be going through life in a continuous state of unrelenting depression.

If their histamine level can be lowered by oral use of the amino acid methionine, by extra calcium by mouth and by the drug phenytoin, then this depression can be relieved. If you or someone you love has these behavior traits, think about getting a doctor on the case. It could make a dramatic difference—and maybe prevent a major tragedy!

High copper levels in the blood and brain can produce depression and paranoia which can lead to suicide or homicide. This condition can be corrected by the use of a supplement of vitamin C with zinc and manganese. The removal of excess copper takes 2 to 3 months, however, so this logical treatment may still not save the patient's life if suicidal tendencies are present.

Those who succeed in committing suicide have a lower level of a serotonin metabolite in their brain fluids. The metabolite is 5-hydroxy indole acetic acid (5-HIAA). Serotonin is a normal neurotransmitter in the brain and its dietary precursor is the essential amino acid tryptophane which may be low in a junk food diet. Tryptophane, in doses of 1 to 2 grams, is used at bedtime to promote normal sleep which occurs when tryptophane is made into serotonin in the brain. Since suicidal states frequently follow severe insomnia, the use of tryptophane for sleep is a logical step in the prevention of suicide.

Any of these biological factors may be present in the person attempting or thinking about suicide. Get yourself or your loved one to a doctor if you have any doubts about your physical or mental health—or your nutritional intake.* If these conditions are diagnosed and corrected, suicidal mood changes dramatically for the better.

Premenstrual Syndrome

The presence of magnesium in chocolate might be the reason many women crave this brown goodie just the day before their periods. This does not indicate a chocolate deficiency; they have a magnesium deficiency.

Premenstrual symptoms include abdominal bloating, weight gain, breast tenderness, irritability, headache, depression, and edema, the water-logged feeling. Sometimes you don't make the association between the fact that you are feeling horribly fat and that in a few days your period is due. Your friends and parents don't consider the fact that your period is due either, when you are crabby one moment and burst into tears the next.

Your susceptibility to stress, allergies, and infections, the resulting headaches, insomnia, and depression, and even your weight gain may be due to the fact that 10 days before your period your blood calcium and zinc and magnesium begin to drop steadily, and your blood copper rises. Taking calcium and magnesium (1,000 mg of each) and vitamin C supplements (1,000 to 5,000 mg) every day for a week before your period (or all the time) might help relieve the tension and depression, and will cut the severity of the cramps.

Vitamin B_6 is needed by the liver to metabolize the female hormone, estrogen. Many women find that extra B_6 along with the calcium and magnesium will get them through their periods with equanimity. If you find yourself weeping unaccountably just prior to your periods, you might try some B_6 (50 to 100 mg a day) and see if the next one is easier and less emotionally devastating. B_6 and zinc (30 to 60 mg a day) can also help establish regular cycles. If your cycles are very irregular, or they stop (and you're not pregnant), this could indicate general malnutrition.

---

* The preceding seven paragraphs were drawn from a personal communication from Lianne Audette and Carl C. Pfeiffer, "Four Biological Factors in Suicide."

I've had dieting female patients whose chief complaint was that their periods did not come. They looked haggard and scrawny as if they had been in a concentration camp. They had little or no reserve fat on their skeletons. When fat reserves get below a set point the hormones that cause ovulation turn off. The thyroid gland slows down, and thyroid hormone is necessary for every cell in the body to function. Premenstrual syndrome is often associated with the yeast infection; candidiasis.

Reducing your consumption of salt and caffeine will have a profound effect on the bloating and breast tenderness that accompany premenstrual syndrome. Remember that cheese, hamburgers, French fries, salted nuts, pretzels, soy sauce, and most junk foods are very high in salt and also in the fats that contribute to the pimples you also get just before your period. It is proven that caffeine and fats affect cysts in the breasts, and these always become tender before menstruation. Cut out coffee, tea, and cola drinks and see what happens. Also try avoiding chocolate, sugar, and sweets for about 10 days before your periods. (Yikes! Just when you are craving them.) Alcohol, especially wine and beer, may increase headaches and cramps. There are some herbal teas, most notably raspberry leaf tea, which might relieve cramps.

If you have heavy menstrual flow you will find that iron supplements are necessary, but get a blood check for anemia occasionally. Vitamin A can slow a heavy flow.

Acne: You Hate to Look in the Mirror Because You Are Covered with Greasy Skin Dotted with Zits

Why is it that when you are so embarrassed about the way you look anyway, you get creamed with pimples on your exposed skin so the whole world can see. It is not fair.

Dermatologists have been trained to state publicly that diet has nothing to do with acne, but you and I know that diet makes a difference. Eat it today and wear it tomorrow. Many dermatologists have told patients of mine that they have to admit that diet can affect the skin. Diet change and nutritional therapy are slow, but they are safer than drug treatment. And a good nutritional approach will allow the orthodox treatment to be more effective.

Acne is a disorder of the oil glands, and it occurs most commonly during adolescence because this is when the hormones which influence the secretion of the oil glands are operating at their peak. Vitamin A at a dosage of 50,000 to 100,000 units a day for a month might make a difference, along with 60 to 90 mg of zinc. If there is some clearing, the dose can be reduced to once a week or whatever seems appropriate. (Big doses of vitamin A can cause headaches, dry mouth, hair loss, and double vision, so stop if any of these things occur, but the dose needs to be high for a while to encourage the formation of dry skin, which is beneficial for the acne control. This is considered a toxic dose by some. If a girl suspects she is pregnant, she should stick to 20,000 units or less. Most can tolerate these big doses for a month without any toxic effects.) Also, the B-complex vitamins, especially riboflavin, pyridoxine, and pantothenic acid, help to reduce oiliness. (Most use a capsule with 25 to 100 mg of each of the B's in it daily.) Vitamin C helps reduce the secondary infection in the oil glands (2,000 to 10,000 mg a day depending on the bowel tolerance), and vitamin E will minimize the scarring (most stick to 800 to 1,200 units a day for a month or two, then cut the dose in half). Vitamin D helps guard the body's store of calcium. Judicious use of ultraviolet light can dry the skin, allow some peeling to open the oil glands up, and control some of the infection.

Psychological stress also seems to be a factor in acne, so all the nutrients needed to meet stress—calcium, magnesium, and the B vitamins—should be emphasized. Calcium also helps to maintain the acid-alkali balance of the blood necessary for a clear complexion.

If you have pimples on your face and white spots on your nails, a zinc deficiency is probably the main cause of your skin condition. However, if you have pimples on your face and pimples on your buttocks and no white spots on your nails, you are more likely dealing with a food sensitivity.

As usual, overindulgence in sugar and fats exacerbates the problem. Cheese, beef, French fries, potato chips, and milk shakes are all very high in fat. Other foods most likely to cause some trouble are cola drinks, whole milk, nuts and seeds (high in fat), some seafood (because of the iodine), and anything else you really like. You should find that becoming a vegetarian or semivegetarian for a while might help to control the eruptions. Vegetables, fruit, whole grains, stream or lake fish, and some organically grown fowl might help smooth out the mess. Cleanliness is worthwhile, of course, but scrubbing the pimples off just increases the damage already inflicted.

You can combine a dietary approach with over-the-counter preparations, but, if you get nowhere, a visit to the dermatologist is a good idea, if only to find out whether the skin doctors have learned anything new. They know that some basic skin defatters and an antibiotic are the standard treatment. But hold it: Antibiotics can be dangerous. They allow yeast infections to grow and allow some resistant germs to flourish. They also mess up your digestive tract; eating lots of yogurt and acidophilus bacteria can set it right. Maybe if both of you think that you need the antibiotic you could compromise and take it for the few days just before a date or some special event. It might not wreck the balance of the good and bad bacteria in your intestinal tract if you can take the antibiotic only intermittently. A new vitamin-A analog, called cis-retinoic acid, has proved helpful for those with the terrible scarring type of acne, called cystic.

Gas, Bloating, and Stomach Cramps

Although intestinal gas is normal and everyone has some, it always seems to break loose at the most embarrassing times. Do you say "Sorry," or is it better to pretend it was someone else when you clear your nether throat?

Doctors of gasology have estimated that most gas comes from swallowed air and people who talk while eating are swallowing the most. Bacterial action on undigested food also accounts for much gas formation. We are all aware of the gas we make after beans, garlic, onions, and cabbage, but if you have a *great* deal of gas (how do you know?), or you think you have more than your friends, it may mean you are eating something to which you are allergic. The list is endless, but the most likely offenders are your favorites: dairy, corn, wheat, soy, eggs, nuts, shellfish. Anything can do anything.

It takes four days of abstinence from a food to test whether it is an offender, except dairy products, which take 3 weeks of abstinence. Always the things you love.

If you frequently eat a food to which you are sensitive, the intestinal lining cells that contain the enzymes of digestion actually atrophy and the food sits there undigested. Intestinal bacteria move on up and attack the food, and much smelly gas is the result—a tough problem on a date or when you are sitting in a windowless classroom. Sometimes methane is produced; lighting a match could be disastrous.

Usually adolescents have plenty of stomach acid and have little trouble digesting meat, which requires this hydrochloric acid to break down the protein. Adults after age 35 make less HCl, so they have some trouble with meat digestion and must cut down on the intake of Big Macs. The minerals calcium, magnesium, iron, zinc, and copper may be absorbed better in an acid medium. Older folk usually need to take supplements to be sure of adequate absorption. Vitamin C will enhance the absorption of the minerals.

If you notice fullness right after eating, it may indicate a food allergy, or that your stomach acid is insufficient to handle the food you just sent down. Betaine hydrochloride might be helpful. (Ask at the health store.) If, however, you have stomach pain in the middle just below your breastbone on an empty stomach and swallowing food makes it go away, it suggests you have too much acid or, rarely at your age, a duodenal ulcer. We were taught 40 years ago to drink milk to neutralize that acid; now the evidence indicates a rebound hypersecretion of acid after the original milk ingestion. Milk may actually cause the ulcers.

Constipation

Does your mother still ask you if you had a bowel movement each day? Some parents were taught that a person must have a BM daily or else he or she would go crazy, or it would back up and cause an obstruction or somehow squash the liver and the heart. We now know that the consistency of the stool is more important than the frequency. If you are eating the proper amount of fiber, you should have one or two soft, large, moist, easy-to-pass bowel movements every day.

There is no doubt that straining at stool leads to varicose veins, hemorrhoids, diverticulitis, and hiatus hernia. Stick to vegetables, fruit, seeds, nuts, whole grains, chicken, and fish. Milk, cheese, ice cream, white bread, and sugar are all devoid of fiber and roughage. By the time these processed foods have moved through your intestinal tract and get to your rectum, you will only have a little dust to pass. Drinking more fluid only makes more urine; there is nothing to hold the moisture in the stools until they pass through. We all need roughage and fiber. A big, hard stool sitting in your pelvis is a heavy stress and drains energy from your brain. Now *that* could make you a little dingy. Don't waste your time in the bathroom.

Muscle Aches

Most of us have had muscle cramps, shin splints, or growing pains, especially after exercising or while growing fast. I am disturbed that doctors do not seem to realize that they are almost always due to lactic acid accumulation—a normal end product of anaerobic metabolism. Calcium seems to be the answer for most of this pain.

If you are drinking milk and you are still having muscle pains, you are probably allergic to cow juice and your intestinal lining cells are poisoned so they cannot absorb the calcium from the milk. Dump it. If you cannot get enough calcium from the good diet recommended by Martha Rose (turnip greens, collards), then you must try 1,000 mg of calcium and 1,000 mg of magnesium daily. If it's winter, some cod-liver oil (400 to 1,000 units) daily would be appropriate. If you have some muscle cramps and some difficulty relaxing and sleeping, the calcium and the magnesium are best taken about an hour before bedtime. I chew mine up along with some unsalted nuts and I can stand the chalky taste (ugh).

Insomnia

The most common cause of trouble falling asleep—sleep resistance—is the inability to relax. The most common cause of the inability to relax is an excess of adrenalin. Adrenalin is secreted by the adrenal glands in times of stress or emotional upheaval—we all know that. You have a test tomorrow, your folks are fighting, your best friend is moving away, anything. But you should also know that things you eat will stimulate the flow of adrenalin. When the blood sugar rises and falls, adrenalin is needed to get sugar out of its storage in the liver and to get the body ready to run or fight.

If you are lying in bed staring at the ceiling feeling ner-

vous—with dry mouth, tingly, sweaty skin, moist palms, rapid
heartbeat, tightness in the stomach—it might mean you ate
something in the last one to four hours to which you are allergic,
or you had some sugar or a soft drink.

But it may also mean that you are not getting enough calcium and magnesium in your diet. We all need them for teeth
and bones, but many of us cannot extract the minerals from the
food we eat because of the poor quality of the food, inadequate
stomach acid, and improper balance of the calcium, magnesium, and phosphorus in the foods. Calcium and magnesium
are necessary for the propagation of nerve impulses. If the supplies of these minerals are inadequate, the receptive part of the
brain notices too many stimuli coming in from the environment;
the brain perceives that the environment is a stress, or, more
exactly, a *dis*tress.

While you are lying there trying to relax, ask yourself where
do you get your calcium and magnesium. Is it all from dairy
products? These sources may be inadequate because of your
allergy to them. Magnesium is in chlorophyl, but are you eating
collards, turnip greens, parsley, and the other related goodies?
Are you spooked by noises? That is a magnesium deficiency. (A
chocolate craving may also mean a magnesium deficiency.)

If you eat a lot of meat and drink sodas, you could be throw-
ing your calcium-phosphorus ratio out of whack, and you will
lose calcium. Blood-sugar fluctuations will cause calcium to run
out of the body.

Whether you have reasons to lie awake worrying or not, you
need the sleep, so take 1,000 mg of calcium (chelated or orotate
are fairly expensive and no better than carbonate or oyster shell)
and 1,000 mg of magnesium (mag oxide works and is cheap)
about an hour before climbing into bed. I assume you are also
trying the menu ideas proposed by Martha Rose.

Some try tryptophan, 500 to 3,000 mg or so, close to bedtime,
as it turns to serotonin in the brain and helps to calm one. You
can make your own serotonin if you eat some carbohydrate,
preferably complex, in the evening. The tryptophan floating
around in the blood stream will get to the brain more easily
because the other amino acids are stored in the tissues when
the insulin level rises after a carbo load.

Caffeine may allow you to get going in the morning and keep
going during the day, but its stimulating effects suggest it

should not be used after noon or so. Remember, there is a lot of caffeine in tea, many soft drinks, and in some cold and cough remedies. I used to drink coffee just before bedtime and it would help me fall asleep. I finally figured that was crazy, and then I realized that I am somewhat hyperactive, and stimulants have a calming effect on those so touched. To each his own. Now I do better if I take calcium and magnesium along with some complex carbohydrate like vegetables or almonds just before bedtime.

Frequent Infections

If you are sick a lot with respiratory, skin, bladder, or intestinal infections, you must be aware by now that going to the doctor is helpful, but antibiotics are just treating the disease. Doctors (M.D.s) rarely delve into the uncharted waters of prevention. "Stay out of drafts, get your eight hours sleep, wear warm dry socks, eat three meals a day, and don't kiss anyone with a cold or mono," is about all they know, and they got that from their mothers—not from medical school.

What you should be aware of is that your immune system is not up to par. It is not normal to be sick, but it is average. The immune system needs protein to make white blood cells, immune globulins, and antibodies. It needs vitamins C, E, A, and the B-complex vitamins. Sugar ingestion will actually paralyze the ability of the white blood cells to phagocytize the bacteria. Stress can weaken the immune system; just your *perception* that the world is stressful is enough to reduce the effectiveness of your defense system. Allergic people are more prone to infection.

Remember, those viruses, bacteria, and fungi are everywhere on your skin, up your nose, down your gullet, just waiting for a break in the surface so they can get a foothold and grow in your juicy tissues. And if you have had antibiotics because of ear, throat, bronchial, or bladder infections, and you have taken tetracycline for your acne, you are a setup for an overgrowth of the yeast in your intestinal tract. That yeast releases a toxin that produces symptoms but also overwhelms the already depleted immune system, causing a weakness that will allow you to get sick again. A vicious cycle.

An infection or flu or sickness is a (slight) blessing, as it tells you that the guards at the gates went to sleep. Vitamin C is the key support for the immune system. All the health gurus suggest this regime to be begun when you are in reasonable health: take 1,000 mg of vitamin C (calcium, magnesium ascorbate is probably the best) the first day. Increase this by 1,000 mg each day until you have reached a dose (5,000 to 10,000 mg a day is the usual amount) that starts to cause some softness of your bowel movements. That is the saturation dose. Cut back the dose to the amount that is just short of this effect; that is the daily prophylactic dose.

When a cold or virus strikes you, don't wait to see if it is Asian flu or mono or the Hoboken quick-step, assume that you need help with your immune system and take the daily dose that you have previously determined every hour until the symptoms have decreased. Most of the time the disease will not develop because the extra ascorbic acid has helped the body manufacture enough interferon, a natural, intracellular, antiviral substance. It also helps the other parts of the immune system do their jobs more easily. The big doses of the C will not cause diarrhea because the body will absorb more C when the need increases; little of the swallowed C will get to the rectum to irritate the nether passage.

Continue the large dose for a day or so until the disease is under control and then gradually reduce the amount and frequency until you get back to the original basic daily dose at the same time that the disease symptoms are eliminated.

If this regime gets you nowhere, get some blood tests to rule out low gamma globulin and poor white blood cell function. Not everything is a nutritional fault.

Halitosis

It is hard to tell if your own breath is offensive to others unless someone tells you. But I can remember when I was 14 to 16 years old how I thought my breath was just awful, like something had died and was hanging there down the back of my throat. I would talk with my hand over my mouth to deflect the effluvium. I tried sprays and mouth washes, had my mouth and throat checked, had the dentist search for pus sequestered in the teeth, put ointments up my nose—but nothing helped. I had to clear my throat every 20 minutes, I had nosebleeds a lot. Somewhere about that time I ran out of milk and the phlegm, the blood, and the stink all disappeared. It was all a milk sensitivity, and it all fit my history of childhood infections in my nose, throat, and ears. I even had to have my mastoid bone reamed out at age 5 years. The milk allergy had been causing the phlegm, or at least had triggered the infections, or the sensitivity to milk made me more susceptible to the infections. Bacteria can create a bad odor.

So if you've brushed your teeth, and your tonsils are not chronically infected, you might consider your diet. And not just the phlegm from the milk but the food that is fermenting or putrefying down in your intestines. The liver is supposed to clear this sludge, but apparently some of it slips by and gets to the lungs and is exhaled onto your friends. Lozenges, sprays, and mints are just a Band-Aid approach.

Vegetarians say they can tell if there are meat-eaters nearby.

Stop eating your favorite food for a few days. Try a cleansing diet of just fruit and vegetables for four days and notice how fresh and clean you become. It takes three weeks, however, for the body to clear itself of the chemicals produced from dairy product ingestion.

The following supplements will promote efficient digestion: vitamins A, C, the B complex (especially B_6, niacin and PABA); magnesium and zinc, chlorophyl, and digestive enzymes. Some find that yogurt and acidophilus are helpful.

Body Odor

BO is a part of being alive and breathing. Some of our body wastes exit through the skin. We should bathe every day or so and change our socks and underwear. I like the sweet smell of a fresh, sweaty body, but the bacteria and fungi on our hair, armpits, and crotch quickly multiply and the odor therefrom is not pleasant. When combined with the increased function of the oil glands that accompanies adolescence, one can become really gamey and persona non grata. The disagreeable odor must be Mother Nature's way of telling us to shower or bathe; if the little nasties growing all over our skin find a portal of entry, we can get boils, carbuncles, paronychia, impetigo, athlete's foot, jungle rot, and crotch itch. The body odor is just a clue that something more serious is possible.

But if you *have* bathed, you *have* powdered and deodorized, and there is still an aura of disgust hanging about you like a shadow, you might look to your diet (as in halitosis). A deficiency of a mineral often lacking in our diet can produce an unwashable, pervasive, heavy, repugnant odor. If all else fails, magnesium deficiency should be considered, especially if you have not been faithful about eating magnesium-laden foods (green vegetables, nuts and seeds). (A low threshold for noises is another sign of a magnesium deficiency.) Try 500 to 1,000 mg of magnesium oxide every day for a month. (Is this why dogs eat grass occasionally? Magnesium is in the chlorophyll molecule.) Some odoriferous people are low in zinc; 30 to 60 mg a day for a month should help. The B complex and chlorophyll might help as well.

Dandruff

It was not until a few years ago (age 40 plus) that I found some nutritional help that would have made by own life easier or at least less embarrassing back in those "what a stupid body" days. I had tried everything the barber suggested for my dandruff, and the degreasers and shampoos and stiff brush treatments helped, but the stuff kept returning. This barber said the dandruff was from washing with hot water. "Did you ever see a bear with dandruff?" I guess that's true; bathing in those cold mountain streams must help.

More recently I realized that milk, cheese, ice cream, and sugary garbage were the biggest cause of my scaly, itchy scalp. I also read that vitamin B_6 was helpful in controlling seborrhea, which is a skin condition related to dandruff and greasy, scaly skin.

I have seen many babies with yellow greasy scales in the hairs of their upper eyelids, behind their ears, and on the soft spot at the top of the head. Some even had a groin rash. Many of them came from mothers who had nausea and vomiting during the first three months of pregnancy. Apparently some people have a genetically determined dependency on certain nutrients (B_6 in this case). Poor dream recall might suggest this possibility. Most of us do not have an out-and-out deficiency.

Vitamin A is not found in the adolescent's diet to any great extent, and the proper dose should make the skin somewhat dry. (See acne.) One could try 20,000 to 50,000 units a day for only three to four weeks, and, if the greasy scales are lessened, could then cut back to 10,000 to 20,000 units a day as a maintenance dose.

Eating greasy hamburgers, french fries, and milk shakes seems to fill up the oil glands as well as the stomach. The oil glands manufacture those scales. One might try vegetarianism for a couple of weeks and see what happens. I get benefit from hair shampoos and conditioners with jojoba in them.

Hair Problems

Since hair is composed chiefly of protein one must make sure that the protein intake is of good quality and adequate. Sulfur-bearing amino acids, as are found in eggs, contain the most efficient hair-makers known. Dull, dry hair may be a sign of a vitamin-A deficiency but is also seen in a vitamin-A overdose. Biotin, folic acid, inositol, pantothenic acid, copper, iodine, and zinc all are needed for proper hair growth. Many with hypothyroidism report that the hair was the first thing to become abnormal and lackluster.

Dry skin and hair can flake and itch. Some people, especially those who are touched with eczema, need to bathe with as little soap as possible (Neutrogena is good). Bath oils are a good idea (Alpha-Keri is a standard). Ordinary soap and water will remove the protective layer of oil from the skin; this is good if you are greasy, but devastating if you are already genetically dry. Soaking in the tub with oil in the water, or putting the oil on as soon as you pat yourself dry, will hold the moisture in the surface cells.

If your hair is stringy and oily, it may be due to the sugar and the fat in your diet. The thing you love to eat is probably the thing causing your whatever.

What to Do If:

You are a male and notice that your breasts are budding.   About 50 percent of males will notice breast buds during puberty. This is due to a normal but short-lived surge of estro-

gen that occurs in the male. It does not mean the young man is
turning into a girl. The condition is transitory. It can be exaggerated with marijuana use.

**You are a male and notice a soft swelling above the
testicle, usually on the left.** This is usually a gathering of
dilated veins carrying blood away from the testicle. About one in
four have this condition, and it has no significance if the testi-
cles are both of equal size. This varicocele may be associated
with atrophy of the testicle in some cases; a doctor should be
consulted.

What to Do If You Are Cold When Others Are Comfortable

You wear socks to bed, you would wear gloves, too, except it
seems silly, you are constipated, tired, sluggish, sleep well but
are never refreshed after sleeping all night.

It is not hibernation; it may be a sluggish thyroid gland. You
would do well with a checkup and blood tests to stumble on an
anemia, hidden infection, or low thyroid function. If the kindly
physician says your body is okay and the tests are normal, and
begins the lecture about the new generation and how it is not
motivated and is downright lazy, thank him or her for all the
trouble and go home to figure yourself out. Do take your morning temperature for five minutes or so in your mouth or your
armpit before you get out of bed. It should be 97.8° to 98.2°. If it
is 96 something up to 97.6°, it suggests the thyroid gland is
working but not well enough for *your* particular body. (An elevated serum cholesterol often accompanies a low thyroid function.) Low thyroid function is often associated with the yeast
infection, candidiasis.

Now, if your temperature is low, you must talk the doctor
into prescribing some thyroid medication. Most of us use desiccated thyroid as it is safer than the synthetic types which may
be more accurate. One grain a day is the way to start. This is
then increased to 2 a day in a week or so if one is still a slug-
abed. You rarely need up to 4 grains and you may not need it for
more than a few months. It may be just the spark you need to
get your body to work properly again.

You may be surprised how your bowels work more easily.

Your eczema may clear, your weight may stabilize, your periods regulate themselves, and you have an all-around good feeling about life. The thyroid hormone is necessary for the function of every cell of the body. If you do not have enough thyroxin flowing about your body, all the motivation and willpower in the world will not get you even close to a suboptimal level of performance.

After a few weeks on the hormone you should notice warmth, comfort, and energy—a good normal feeling. You can even handle stress. Some troublemaker calls you a "jerk," and you say, "Hey, be my guest!" It's fun to be in control. You may find that in a few months you can lower the dose and get off the thyroid medicine. It is as if you have gotten the car going on a cold day and now it can run on its own.

What's Wrong with Me?

"Everybody else seems to be having such a swell time. They all seem to be so perfect, thin, good-looking, and healthy. They don't have skin trouble. They're good athletes or popular. What happened to me?"

There is no way you can live inside another person's body and feel his or her emotions, think his or her thoughts, and notice his or her body symptoms. I thought back there when I was 16 years old that I was the only one who was suffering. All my friends looked like Mr. Cool to me and I felt I was the klutz. My body would not do the things my mind thought up. My pimples turned to ugly open sores that had to scab over before they would heal. My thighs used to rub together like hot dogs stuffed with fat when I walked. I had few muscles that I could see. My nose would bleed if I laughed or cried too vigorously. I had bad breath, sweaty palms, and smelly feet. I knew that everyone was laughing at me and my stupid, noncompliant body. What a mixture of contrasting feelings!

It was not until I began to have adolescent patients in my medical practice who would confide in me some of their fears and anxieties that I finally realized that that poor slob (me) had not been alone back there. Everyone growing up has serious thoughts about the way they are turning out, and even in the best home with the most supportive parents adolescents feel they are dumb, oafish, and not worthy.

Those other kids out there that you so admire and would want to imitate are having just as much trouble holding themselves together as you are. They have fears and phobias that are so illogical they are afraid to share them with you because you might laugh. (How about the myth of growing hair on the palm of your hand if you masturbate? Whom do you ask to find out if it is true or not?)

We need more communication between teens and adults—nonjudgmental adults, that is. I know some outstanding pediatricians who welcome this interchange with the patients; after all, they have been watching their patients growing over the last decade or so, just like the parents. But if you sense that your pediatrician is upset by your incipient pubic hair and he or she suggests by word or action that the maturing adolescent embarrasses him or her, then it's time to find another doctor. That pediatrician probably went into pediatrics in the first place so to avoid having to face the adult body.

You could ask your doctor some simple, wide-open question like, "Do you believe adolescents should get an allowance for making their beds and cleaning up their rooms?" If the doctor's face gets stern and he or she snaps off some absolute rules, and otherwise acts like a dictator, maybe you'd better not ask other personal questions. What you want is someone to whom you can speak about your innermost feelings and fears and some of your crazy ideas without fear that they will laugh in your face or run about the neighborhood telling everyone what you said in confidence.

Meanwhile, try to build your body and mind so that you are at your maximum potential at all times. There is no way you can do this without adhering to some basic health rules. Diet is the most obvious place to begin. Eat simple, fresh foods in small amounts at frequent intervals; exercise regularly. You will maintain your ideal weight more effectively and consistently, and your peace of mind will be more even too.

CHAPTER 3

Self-Image, Bulimia, and Anorexia

TO THE TEENAGER: If I were a young adolescent and began to realize that my body was not turning out as ideally as I'd thought it would, I would be discouraged, at the least, and most probably depressed. "I am going to live in this stupid body all the rest of my life; no trade-ins allowed. Nothing seems to be going right. My parents only speak to me if I have not cleaned up my room; my friends avoid me because I'm fat or klutzy or both. School work is a drag. What's the point?"

If everything is going splendidly, if you are having fun, doing well in school or in sports, in drama or computers, or you are cheerleading or have a boyfriend to be excited about, you may not think too much about how your body looks—either to yourself or to the world. If a girl arrives at puberty with a decent self-image, and notices that her body is not exactly Miss America material, she is well equipped to accept this with equanimity and good humor. "I'm okay; so big deal!"

Are you comfortable most of the time? Do you laugh and smile more than you cry and frown? If you can answer "yes" to these queries, then your self-image is probably satisfactory. Doctors of internal medicine have told me that if their patients are comfortable and satisfied with their lives more than 60 percent of the time, then they are probably doing as well as can be expected.

A positive self-image seems to be a prerequisite for dealing well with the difficult teenage time of life (and for any stressful time, for that matter). Your parents probably helped load you up with enough of that to last a lifetime when you were a cute, smiling infant, loving you and cuddling and accepting you.

The problem is, all the loving and affection parents can give their child can't compete with all the other stimuli—like television and advertising—that affect teens' self-image. A recent study by *Self* magazine (October 1984) shows that, supportive parents, relatives, and friends notwithstanding, more than 50 percent of women under the age of 21 would like to change their legs and thighs. The percentage drops to about 30 percent by the age of 40, after they've had a couple of decades to "get used to" their bodies. Even this percentage looks sadly high to me.

The *Self* magazine article went on to say that the various media are unrealistic in suggesting an impossible ideal figure for all women. This is unattainable for most women, and the efforts that so many make to achieve it are usually unhealthy and even dangerous.

Most women who feel they are too fat have talked themselves into believing that men won't look at a woman with rounded thighs. If these young women would think about pleasing themselves first, and not trying to meet what they think the male specifications are, they would be a much healthier, happier group.

But the media cannot be blamed for everything. Some of the pressure comes from the peer group, an adolescent's "home away from home." For you, a teenager, your peer group is the support organization that gives you a sense of validity; it is a source of constant assessment. You need to feel that you are not too different from your chosen friends, and if you feel that your body does not measure up to the group's standards, you will not get that sense of reassurance. Girls reinforce the feeling in each other that they need to lose weight, and boys feel like they need to gain or grow, or at least have more muscles showing.

I thought the bodybuilding club John and I organized at age 13 would really do it—until I fell asleep under the sunlamp. It's hard to look cool, svelte, and be clever with pink, painful skin. It's best to be yourself. If you have big shoulders and a tapering waist, flaunt it. (Weightlifting and exercise can help you get that look.) But if you are built like a size-40 scorpion, maybe a career in the arts would be more appropriate. Be reasonable; be sensible. Do the best with the body you have inherited.

If you suspect your self-image could be better, there are some things you can do yourself to improve your attitude without resorting to psychotherapy. We know that everyone has some interest, skill, or talent. You may not know that you have it until you experiment a little. I was so bad at sports my folks got me into stamp collecting; I couldn't lose. I'd put a stamp in the right space and Mom would say, "Great."

How about trying the chess club, the speaking or debating team, the history club, the drama group? Sign up for community service at the local hospital or nursing home. Learn to play an instrument. I know a woman who decided no one had made a definitive investigation on the earthworm. She did. She is now a world-recognized expert. She does not care if she is overweight or not. She felt good about herself and her accomplishment. (But how does one bring up the subject at a dinner party?)

TO THE PARENT: It is difficult for most adults to project ourselves back to our adolescence and remember what method we used as our unique style of rebellion. I pouted. My brother bought a motorcycle. Some let their hair grow. Some of you probably wore clothes your parents thought unacceptable. Many youths use food as a weapon, possibly triggered by their parents insistence on "Finish your plate," "Time to eat. I mean now!" "You should eat at least one bite of broccoli." The rule: Your child will defy you in your cherished area; if you are neat, he will be sloppy. If you like verbal and open communication, she will be sullen and silent. This growing personality is finding some autonomy by making a statement to test the limits. The confrontation is staring you in the face.

Food is such an integral part of family life that it is easy to use it as a focus of rebellion. There are many forms of eating disorders, some temporary and innocent—like putting salsa on everything—while others, including bulimia and anorexia, are serious and usually need professional help. Most disorders, fortunately, are somewhere on the milder side of these two nasty entities. One episode of vomiting does not make a disease.

Bingeing and Purging: Bulimia

So the youngster with the feeble self-image arrives at adolescence with the wrong body—the body that doesn't seem to be able to tell the brain when enough calories have been swallowed to just keep even with the ideal weight and optimum energy. Depression sets in and he or she figures, "What the hell," and scarfs down 5,000 to 30,000 calories in about 30 minutes. The stress of a negative perception of the world pushes the blood sugar down and the self-control department of the brain is not operative. The foraging instinct is set in motion. When the victim realizes he or she has no self-control, guilt sets in and the "I'm no good" center makes everything look pretty black.

A full stomach and slight nausea suggests vomiting might provide relief; she gags herself, vomits; the distention disappears. She has discovered control. What a great feeling! What a way to manage weight, enjoy food, and have a degree of control over her life! Bingeing and vomiting (or purging) are easy but costly ways of attempting to establish personal autonomy. It is one way of solving the struggle with food, which many adolescents consider their greatest enemy. But it is not normal and it's very dangerous; it allows the participant to disregard body clues that are supposed to be used to modify eating habits.

People are supposed to eat, become comfortably satisfied, and then quit. All sorts of internal neuro-endocrine mechanisms are set into motion when it is time to eat, when the blood sugar falls, or when one smells or sees food. These are the natural signals that initiate "foraging." If the proper foods for that particular body are swallowed, the mechanisms for ending the eating behavior are flicked on.

But if high-calorie, low-nutrient foods are consumed, these

built-in clues cease to operate. The *amount* of food swallowed is one limiting factor, but by the time the information gets to the satiety center in the brain, more calories than needed have been consumed and weight gain can result. The secret to weight and energy control is to eat foods that are filling but, at the same time, release their calories over a long period of time, foods like whole grains and vegetables and some fruits and nuts (as opposed to simple sugar or refined carbohydrates, i.e., junk food). Hence the pancreas is not stimulated to squirt out large amounts of insulin which would push the blood sugar down and set up the craving for a quick sugary fix.

When you eat calorie-dense foods that make your blood sugar rise and fall rapidly, the bingeing pattern of overeating can be set in motion because (1) you're hungry and (2) your low blood sugar and the direct effect that a rapidly rising level of insulin has on the brain prevents the brain from functioning in a social way; judgment and self-control are gone.

When judgment and self-control slip, the victim may become mean and surly. Some fall into depression, and if the self-image is feeble to begin with, this tendency will be overwhelming and bulimia might become established.

The point of all this is that if one has a poor self-concept, he or she may survive through a stressful adolescence. But if falling blood sugar triggers a genetic depressive tendency in this already tilted person, a tough disease may be set in motion.

Bingeing is episodic overeating. If one gains weight, it is called too much overeating. If overeating leads to self-induced vomiting or swallowing a laxative (purging) to rid oneself of the caloric load, it is called bulimia. It is a condition which has reached epidemic proportions among teenagers in our country. Most bulimics are in the normal weight range for their height.

The bulimic is a victim of intertwining psychological, genetic, environmental, and biochemical forces. If one has a poor self-image to begin with and one regards eating as gluttony, the psychological implications seem obvious: swallowing one Twinkie is stepping over the line; self-loathing, despair, and loss of control follow. "I'm bad; I might as well eat a dozen now." As alcoholics know, one drink is too many and a thousand are not enough. But the psychological motivations for bingeing are insignificant when the biochemistry of the foraging center takes over.

Sugar-cravers must understand that they overproduce insulin when they eat sugary foods or eat foods to which they are allergic. When the blood sugar falls, they lose control. *They don't lose control because they are bad people.* It is not a moral question. Given their biochemical situation, it is almost natural for them to binge. And then, to relieve the situation and to regain a sense of control, they induce vomiting (or they purge).

Bingeing and purging have been known throughout history, but have reached pathological proportions only in the last four decades, and only in our country (although the condition exists in other modern, fashion-conscious countries, like Italy and France). I believe that it is related more to biochemistry than to psychology. That is why we have developed so many recipes in this book designed to keep the blood sugar at a good functioning level, sufficient to prevent the drop that triggers the foraging center.

Once the bulimic is into the binge-purge cycle, chemistry reinforces the procedure. Biochemists tell us that vomiting releases endorphins and allows one to cope, as do drugs or exercise. (Starvation will release endorphins also.) A carbohydrate load tends to allow tryptophan to get to the brain which promotes serotonin manufacture. The latter has a calming effect. A temporary way out becomes a way of life. The corollary with alcoholism is obvious.

About a third of the people with eating disorders seem to have addictive personalities: many also abuse alcohol, cigarettes, and drugs. They need help. When a magazine article appeared a few years ago about the problem, the editorial offices were flooded with calls and letters begging for help. These women were so delighted to find others paralyzed with this pervasive problem, their own private hell of self-imposed isolation.

Bulimics usually have a normal drive to maintain a decent weight, look trim, enjoy food, and have some control over their bodies. These people (80 to 90 percent are women) are action-oriented, busy joiners, socially involved, and, as adults, often are married, have children and a career. Bulimia is a very lonely, secret condition, and it is amazing to find that bulimics have kept this "secret" from their families for years. Psychotherapists tell us that these patients, when they finally come to them for help, are surprised and relieved to find that thousands of other "normal" people are locked into this compulsive, agonizing routine.

Eating disorders, including bulimia and anorexia, are sometimes associated with depression. One study indicated that there was a high, positive relationship of family history of depression in patients with bulimia and anorexia.[1] No one knows whether depression leads to eating disorders or vice versa; if you are depressed, you usually eat less—but you might eat more. If you eat nutrient-poor foods, sugary foods, or foods to which you are allergic, you may get depressed. If you overeat junk food, you may get depressed because you have no self-control. Learning difficulties can lead to depression and that could lead to eating disorders. So the idea is to eat well enough so you don't get depressed. And if your brain is well served with good food, you may do better academically.[2] If you have school phobia, it suggests you have a "masked depression."

Many doctors like to treat depression with drugs. Drugs may be okay, but they only treat the symptoms. A physician prescribing drugs usually doesn't consider that nutrition might explain some or all of these symptoms (although many doctors are becoming more and more aware of nutritional science). Remember, the brain cannot have a rash or a gas attack; it is only able to have disturbances in thought, perception, and feeling. These brain functions are determined by neurotransmitters, and they are made by enzymes, and enzymes need energy, vitamins, and minerals. Even Hippocrates said, "Let your food be your medicine."

We were taught in medical school that if a person had an eating disorder—too thin, too fat, just right but eats and vomits, hates food, loves food, has cravings for certain foods, eats wood, paper, dirt—all of these conditions and attitudes were psychiat-

[1] R. L. Hendren, "Depression in Anorexia Nervosa," *Journal of the American Academy of Child Psychiatry,* 22:59 (1983).
[2] W. A. Weinberg et al., "Depression in Children," *Journal of Pediatrics,* 83:1065 (1973).

ric distortions or responses to depression, frustration, anger, or a sense of a loss of autonomy. Supposedly a psychiatrist, or maybe a psychologist, is capable of dealing with these victual victims. Well, we waited and waited for mental health professionals to develop some kind of sensible theory of causation and therapy that was at least 75 percent reliable. This hasn't happened, and few people—or physicians—ever considered diet a possible factor until recently.

Along with the biochemical forces which act on the bulimic, genetic factors (high incidence of alcoholism, obesity, and depression in close relatives) and family influences are closely tied in. There are consistent patterns which have been observed in families of people with eating disorders. Many of them are very strict, maintaining rigid control over activity, emotions, and even thoughts. Perfectionism runs high; there is a lot of push for achievement, with emphasis on performance, and, often, on physical beauty, thinness, and athletic prowess. With all this pressure, no wonder many of the children grow up angry and depressed. No one can measure up to the kinds of expectations set by these families.

Many families whose children end up with food-related difficulties refuse to express their emotions; they never show their anger or depression. "What would the neighbors think?" Emphasis is on putting on a happy face and loving all family members and friends and pets at all times, no matter how they really feel. Even when their children attain the goals they are pushed so hard to achieve, these parents rarely display pleasure or joy, or even encouragement. They insist on retaining habitual methods of interacting with each other, despite the fact that these methods are counterproductive. If issues try to arise that threaten to force changes—especially about individual autonomy—their verbalizations or actions are suppressed. Religion is sometimes used as a rationale for avoiding conflict: "We should be nice to one another. . . . Turn the other cheek. . . . You should honor your parents. . . ." The male autocrat at the breakfast table who says, "We never allow quarreling at the table" may soon find he is eating alone. Rarely are the children in ·these families encouraged or praised when they have achieved something, anything.

Fathers of bulimics have been found to be distant, maladjusted, immature, easily frustrated, and likely to be alcoholic, with little self-control. Many parents of bulimics have been sick, indifferent, moody, or angry when the children were growing up.

What kind of people are the bulimics? When they were younger they were more likely to have been the hellions, prone to fighting, bad moods, and tears; the rebels the parents tried to tame. If they were chubby, they were aware of it and self-conscious about it. Ellen Schor[3] summarizes the bulimic woman as (usually) having "within her a raging, screaming child that had to steal love because her emotions were not readily acceptable and her needs were not really heard." But you would be hard-pressed to identify most bulimics, because they put so much energy into hiding their condition, to appearing "normal," and they are usually the achievers their parents trained them to be.

The writers and therapists all seem to believe these people are seeking *control*. Controlling the amount and type of food that is going in and coming out seems to be the only bodily function left for them. Everyone needs some sense of autonomy over their life, or stress becomes *dis*stress. For the person with an eating disorder, the eating process becomes the focus in the struggle for control and identity.

Bulimics are generally afraid of food and see hunger as something that must be given in to. With their poor impulse control they fluctuate between indulgence and penance. Ninety percent of their waking hours are devoted to thinking about food. When food cravings strike, the options they see are: (1) Give up and get fat; (2) Stop eating altogether (become anorectic); or (3) Learn how to vomit. They choose the third.

Pediatricians see the same intertwining emotional and biochemical forces at work in bulimics that they see in hyperactive children: a strong need to win, lots of energy, dissatisfaction, mood swings, sensitivity, keen responsiveness to stress, and a constant search for approval. A high percentage of hyperactive children come from families full of diabetes, alcoholism, and obesity. They have a sugar problem, along with a sensitivity to

[3] Ellen Schor, in Janice M. Cauwels, *Bulimia: The Binge-Purge Compulsion* (New York: Doubleday, 1983).

sugar and many foods: milk, chocolate, wheat, corn, soy—whatever they like. They are also deficient in zinc, manganese, molybdenum, selenium, and chromium.

I have been giving bulimics B-complex vitamin injections every day or two if the oral route does not seem to work. Avoiding stress would be a good plan, but many adolescents seem to put themselves into situations where stress seems automatic and adolescence is itself a naturally stressful time. Too many courses, too many dates, too many phone calls, too many sports, too many hobbies, too many boyfriends and girlfriends to juggle, etc. It seems to be an age for testing the limits.

TO THE TEENAGER: Headaches, fatigue, rashes, flu, stomach aches, and a nasty case of mono should be clues that your body's ability to cope has been exceeded. You might be able to handle the crossing over to adulthood if you do not jeopardize your health by eating nutrient-poor foods that cause your blood sugar to plummet. If you have tried the general diet ideas in this book and still cannot resist those cravings for sugar, fat, salt, and junk foods, you might consult with your doctor about a series of B-vitamin injections that might reestablish enzyme function in your gut, liver, and brain, and facilitate self-control. (Two shots a week for three weeks of most any kind of injectable B-complex solution should tell if it is worthwhile: 1 cc intramuscularly. They are safe, but they sting.)

Jane Anne Slochower suggests[4] that obese people eat in response to emotional states such as anxiety or depression. Try this scenario: a friend does not say hello to you, and this is stressful, so your adrenal glands are stimulated, anxiety wells up from inside, blood sugar falls, calcium, magnesium, and B-complex vitamins, especially B_1, run out in the urine. When the blood sugar drops, the self-control region of your brain does not function optimally and the foraging center is activated. All resolve is unavailable for recall and you reach for your favorite quick-energy foods. Blood sugar shoots up and the cycle of bingeing and purging may begin.

[4] Joyce Anne Slochower, Ph.D., *Excessive Eating* (New York: Human Sciences Press, 1983).

"Normal" people eat in response to internal hunger cues. If we could help the excess eaters reduce anxiety and achieve pleasure by some other route, perhaps they would not have to depend on vomiting or purging for weight-control. Anyone who eats should be able to determine if he is eating in response to inner cues, like hunger and the brain's foraging signal, or if he is eating because of stress.

I saw a 30-year-old man the other day whose story should help to illustrate how stress and biochemistry can combine to devastate the body. As a child he had had ear infections and needed a tonsilectomy, because of a milk allergy. Five years ago he was badly injured in a fall. He lost his job and his interest in life. He sat staring into space for a year, gained 100 pounds, and began to drink heavily. Severe hay fever began two years ago. A few months ago he weighed 300 pounds from a diet of beef, dairy products, sugar, and booze, developed a bleeding disease (low platelets), and had to have his spleen removed. He was placed on huge doses of cortisone.

He is now sorting out his life. I am giving him oral, intramuscular, and intravenous vitamin C, calcium, magnesium, and the B complex to rekindle his failed adrenals and enzyme systems. He is off the alcohol, the dairy foods, and the sugar. He is nibbling on vegetables, whole grains, some fruit, and low-fat protein. He has lost 10 pounds in as many days. He has never felt so good as he does now.

The stress of the accident plus the wrong foods allowed him to come down with a genetically programmed illness. His body was trying to get his attention by giving him allergies. When that did not tell him to improve his lifestyle, the body went one more step and gave him idiopathic thrombocytopenic purpura. He was rude to his body; his body finally gave up. The form of the disease is largely genetically determined; the reason for the appearance of the disease is usually based on faulty diets and lifestyles. Some one else would get migraine, or eczema, or colitis. Bulimia might be an end point for others. What is your Achilles heel?

Bulimics need to find therapists they can trust; the therapist cannot show disgust at what the bulimic person is saying or doing. Therapy is aimed at improving self-esteem and helping patients learn to cope with stress. Bulimics need to learn new ways to feel secure, confident, relaxed, and in control. They must learn to trust their own judgment; they need to know that they can eat a normal meal and not gorge, not have to throw up; and that they can maintain a normal weight by eating the right foods, which will keep their blood sugar even, so they won't get those junk food cravings that mark the beginning of the binge-purge cycle.

Here follows a few of the sad but insightful verbalizations these bulimics have given us:

"I was Miss Perfect, so drugs and booze were out; food was always there."

"I never felt at home. Dad was always so distant. I tried to be better, but he was unable to give me any emotional support."

"I was a fat child, but got good grades and played the violin. I was jealous of my older sister who had a perfect figure, but when she became a severe alcoholic, I developed more self-control. I would relax with food. I felt full one night, threw up, and realized I had a method of control."

"Men usually compete by doing—the most, the best, the strongest. Women often compete on the grounds of physical attractiveness. And approval in most of their minds depends on thinness."

"I need love and approval; I also need success. None of these will come my way if I am fat."

"Thinness promises success, admiration, self-sufficiency, everything the women's movement has suggested should go to females. But women's liberation should give support to women by allowing them to weigh what their bodies should weigh."

"Ten years of my life down the toilet along with $20,000 worth of junk food and stomach acid. I lived a lie. I needed rescuing but I was too embarrassed to confess even to a doctor. All that time looking for a place to vomit before the food was absorbed."

"My teeth had to be capped three times in five years because the stomach acid eroded the enamel off."

As with any addiction, at the beginning the need is so strong that you can't imagine the dangers involved, like losing the enamel from your teeth, or becoming obsessed. Since most eating disorders begin during adolescence, I hope you will reread these quotes and seek help if you are becoming one of the victims.

Anorexia Nervosa

Another eating disorder is anorexia nervosa. It was described centuries ago but only became "popular," or at least common, recently. With many it starts out as a quiet determination to lose a few unneeded pounds, but soon becomes a full-blown disease. With others it stems from a negative attitude, conscious or unconscious: "I do not want to mature and tackle the responsibilities that go with adulthood." These young females (90 percent of the victims are women) see their hips and breasts growing larger almost overnight; these changes and accompanying hormones are frightening. At that tender age, they do not feel they can cope with those sweaty-palmed boys leering and even pinching them. It is safer to remain a little girl. They perceive the fat stored under the skin. They decide to stop eating so they will have no fat pads, no breasts, and no menstrual periods.

The experts studying this form of passive-aggression all seem to agree that the youth is trying to effect some control over her life. The noneater perceives herself as locked into a pattern of daily routine by her parents, her school, the world. She has lost her autonomy and feels controlled, helpless, dependent and incompetent.

Anorectics pursue thinness because it represents idealism, goodness, and perfection. "I am in charge," they seem to be saying to the world. To them fat is equated with greed; greed suggests there has been a loss of control.

"The pursuit of thinness is the final step in this [the anorectic's] effort . . . [to achieve] a sense of identity and effectiveness."[4] But the poor anorectic starves herself to the point of poor

[4] Hilda Bruch, cited in Peter Dolly and Joan Gomez, *Anorexia Nervosa* (London: William Heinemann Medical Books, 1979).

judgment. What begins as a seemingly innocent effort to lose
weight (40 percent were fat before the fasting began), with family approval, snowballs; the anorectic becomes emaciated. It becomes apparent that the psychological motives behind the dieting are more complicated than a mere desire to lose weight. The
dieter seems unable to stop herself from starving, and biochemical and nutritional deficiencies take over. Perceptions are affected; the anorectic perceives herself as fat, although everyone
around her sees that she is skin and bones. A small lettuce leaf
and a tablespoon of cottage cheese are a big meal.

Anorexia nervosa is more likely to develop in the upper social groups; in conscientious, obsessive types. They have rou-
tines and rituals. Rebellion is confined to the meal table. It is
difficult for the parents to understand what is happening as this
child has always been ideal—obedient, compliant, and hard-
working. Suddenly, one night at supper the child stops eating.

The mother cajoles, "You must eat something, dear."

The 13-year-old responds, "I feel full." This after one bite of
chicken, six peas, and a tablespoon of potatoes.

Father knows how to handle this, "Damn it, you eat or I
shove it down your stupid throat." He tries. She vomits. Mother
intervenes to calm the scene. The family cannot achieve any
effective intervention because each member is a part of the
disease. The conflict cannot be resolved readily; a psychiatric
and nutritional program is necessary.

Several intertwining patterns are at play in the families of
many anorectic children. The child is enmeshed like a fly that is
caught in the spider's web. She cannot develop a sense of self
because of her emotional ties to her family. In a healthy family
the child is given some choices in the transaction with other
family members and develops a sense of self—of independence
and of autonomy—while at the same time maintaining a sense
of belonging to a unit.

If the family is too rigid to accommodate the child's drive for
independence because this would crack the unyielding structure, the child rebels; the anorectic does this via eating. Many
parents cannot understand the extreme fluctuations of emotions so typical of the "normal" adolescent; closeness and shar-
ing will alternate with overt rejection of one or both parents.

These young people usually wind up in the psychiatrist's office, but the healing process requires time, and the whole family must be involved as attitude changes are necessary. Nutrition plays a large role in therapy. I have seen some anorectic adolescents recover with vitamin shots. Zinc deficiency has been reported in them, because without this trace mineral the taste buds will not function and a dysgeusia, or distorted taste sensation, develops in just a few weeks time. Food may taste like excrement and, obviously, that would make fasting easier. An occasional patient will begin to eat again when diagnosed and treated for an intestinal yeast infection (nystatin is often used to control intestinal candidiasis).

I believe that many people who have fasted for long periods of time can suffer a permanent disruption of the function of the enzymes in the lining cells of the intestinal tract. Once one is sick it is hard to get well; you have to be healthy to be healthy. When those cells are sloughed off because of diarrhea or purging or prolonged eating of nutrient-poor foods, swallowing good foods may not correct the malabsorption. The enzymes responsible for the digestion and absorption of the foods and their associated vitamins and minerals need the vitamins and minerals to accomplish the job. They cannot absorb the vitamins without the vitamins; a catch-22. These situations create the need for the vitamin-B shots; the B complex travels via the circulation to the intestinal lining cells and encourages the enzymes to do what they are supposed to do.

Boys are not usually affected with anorexia, but they are just as concerned as girls with their image. They usually want to be big, muscular, and *macho*—in general. With the proper diet and the appropriate exercise they should be able to achieve the maximum with their physical endowments.

CHAPTER 4

Snacking, Pigging Out, and Bingeing

According to teenagers' reports, there are three types of nonmeal eating: snacking, pigging out, and bingeing. *Snacking* is often done after school and after dinner, alone or with friends, and does not necessarily imply excessive eating (although the food is usually excessively caloric). *Pigging out* is a planned social event. A group of friends gets together, usually on weekends, and eats all day. Eighty percent of teenagers pig out with friends. It is fun, organized, excessive eating, a celebration of the weekend, a way to let go, and a way to rebel. *Bingeing* is not fun; it is usually done alone, when one is feeling empty and out of control. It always ends in feelings of guilt and low self-esteem, as we saw in the previous chapter.

Twenty-five percent of the calories teenagers consume come from snacking. Most snacking is done after school because the teen's hunger is often ravenous, but it could also be the result of boredom or depression. (When snacking alone gets out of hand it becomes a binge.) This is especially true with younger teens, who are expected to go home after school and who find the transition from school to home (where they are often alone) difficult. They come home to an empty house, turn on the television or do their homework, and eat. If there is no ready-to-eat food in the refrigerator or cupboard, they might stop at the corner grocery store on their way home. Older teens often snack in order to keep going through the day, because they don't eat properly. Sugar snacks give them the buzz they need. Snacking in fast food restaurants is often a social event among older teens.

The kind of food kids snack and pig out on is food that is handy and portable. Grocery stores and fast food establishments thrive on these habits. According to a recent survey done in the Bay Area of California, the following list represents, in the order of preference, teenagers' favorite snacks:

candy	peanut butter and jelly sandwich
chocolate	milk
sodas	chicken
chips	nuts
ice cream	cookies
pizza	pastries
fruit	popcorn
fruit juice	burritos
carrots	fries
toast	bagels
Chinese food	burgers
chocolate milk	cereal

Almost all of the foods in this list can be approximated by other foods which have more food value. Teenagers cannot realistically be expected to avoid snacking, but they can at least replace the empty calories with nutritious ones, without sacrificing the flavors they crave. The foods for snacking should be as nutritious as possible. Good foods will be filling and prevent the drop in blood sugar that causes the excess snacking that might eventually evolve into bingeing. Later on in this chapter we will list nutritious equivalents for most of the above foods; they are available at natural food stores and many supermarkets, where more and more space is being devoted to healthy snacks. You will also find easy-to-follow recipes.

How to Control Snacking

TO THE TEENAGER: The underlying mechanism forcing you to eat is falling blood sugar (see Chapter 2). The rule you must remember is to eat foods that provide long-term energy (that is, protein and complex carbohydrates). Vegetables, nuts, seeds, and whole grains are slowly digested in the intestinal tract and the sugars that they finally produce are only slowly, evenly, and gently providing an energy source. Hence the pancreas is not stimulated to squirt out large amounts of insulin which would push the blood sugar down and set up the craving for a quick sugary fix.

Snacking can be the result of hunger; the feeling of an empty stomach can accompany that desire to munch, but not necessarily. When snacking is the result of hunger it means that the meals you are eating are inadequate. If you begin to eat more complex carbohydrates, you will notice less frequent hunger attacks.

Unfortunately, the foods you snack on are so available and visible that sheer willpower can hardly suffice as a means to avoid them; nobody could be expected to have that much resistance. But if you begin to use a little forethought and self-examination you might get some perspective on your snacking. There are things you can do that will help you control the habit.

Are You Hungry?

When you are about to begin your daily snacking ritual, chew on a raw carrot or a little popcorn and ask yourself *why* you want to eat. Are you hungry, *OR*

- bored?
- lonely (or bored *and* lonely)?
- tired?
- tense, so you feel like eating to relax?
- angry at somebody? (Whom? Why?)
- anxious about something? (What?) .
- feeling worthless?
- depressed or upset? (About what?)
- happy? (About what?)

- trying to avoid an unpleasant task (such as homework or house chores)?
- trying to avoid an unpleasant confrontation (with parents, brothers or sisters, friend, boyfriend, or girlfriend)?
- feeling like you need a reward?
- going along with the crowd, which is going to a fast food joint?
- going along with the crowd, which has just ordered a delivery of pizza and shakes?
- trying to forget about a romance that didn't work?
- tempted by the food commercials which you've just seen on television?
- at the movies, where you *always* have candy and a coke?
- at the shopping mall, where there are so many ice cream and fast food places that you can't resist?
- craving a snack because of the smell of something your mother is baking?
- just having this inexplicable craving for something sweet and creamy, or salty and crunchy, and you can't get it out of your head?

Replace Snacking with Another Activity

Having examined the situation and having eaten some long-acting, complex carbohydrate, you now know that you aren't really hungry; but that doesn't keep you from wanting to open a bag of potato chips. The next step is to devise a list of activities which will replace snacking. You can avoid eating by filling your time with something else.

Instead of eating, try one of these activities while you're watching television:

- Do some kind of handwork (knitting, needlepoint, macrame, mending).
- Play computer games.
- Assemble a jigsaw puzzle.

- Prepare vegetables for meals and snacks (see Chapter 11).
- Iron or sort the laundry.
- Draw or paint.
- Work on your scrapbook.
- Do exercises: sit-ups, leg lifts, etc. This might also be the perfect time of day to get your aerobic exercise (see Chapter 8). If you exercise during the time when you normally snack because there's nothing else to do, you will be killing two birds with one stone. It will be less depressing to come home to an empty house if you know that you are going to come home, change right into your running clothes, and go for a jog. If you and your friends normally eat after school, you could all exercise together. Exercising can be a social event just like eating. Usually exercise reduces your appetite, so that you won't be hungry until dinner. You could also exercise an hour after dinner, another time teenagers often find themselves opening the refrigerator door so that they can munch while they do their homework or watch television. Exercise is one of the best ways to deal with tension or depression; you just feel so good afterward, certainly better than you'd feel after eating a bag of potato chips.
- Take a nap. Sometimes you want to snack because you're actually tired. A rest would do the trick better than a sugary nothing.
- Take a walk or a bicycle ride. Getting outside, breathing fresh air, will not only take you away from the kitchen, but it will take your mind away from food.
- Walk the dog.
- Give the dog a bath.
- Call a friend.
- Get together with friends to prepare food.
- Take a shower or a long, hot bath.
- Practice the piano.

- Listen to music; dance.
- Sew.
- Wash the car.
- Clean your room.
- Rearrange your closet (you've been meaning to go through your old clothes forever; now is the time).
- Do something else you've been putting off.
- If you're with friends, do makeovers or give each other haircuts.
- Do your nails.
- Write in your diary.
- Write a letter.
- Read.
- Make some of the healthy snacks in this book.

Keeping a Snacking Notebook

Since eating between meals has more to do with behavior than with hunger, modifying your behavior patterns is the best way to deal with snacking. The first thing to do is to get in touch with your eating behavior, and a good way to begin this is by keeping an eating notebook, in which you note down every time you want to eat, and the accompanying circumstances. Using the format below, record all the times you get the munchies, how you feel at the time, what you crave, etc. If you start taking notes every time you get the urge to eat, you'll not only learn a lot about yourself, but you'll also begin to alter your snacking habits. Just writing all these things down will eventually alter your desire to eat (especially if you are overeating; seeing the candy bars add up on your list may shock you out of eating so many). And even if it doesn't do that much, it will help you replace unhealthy snacks with nutritious ones. Just thinking about all these things helps, and writing them down helps more. Try the notebook for two weeks and let me know.

SNACKING NOTEBOOK

Date: April 14, 1986

Time of Day: 4:00 P.M.

Where: Home, in TV room

Activity at the Time: Watching television

Mood: Feeling empty, alone, depressed, and bored

Whom with: Alone

When did I last eat? Lunch

What did I last eat? Tunafish sandwich, apple, cookie

When is next meal? Dinner, 6:00 P.M.

Degree of hunger (0–3): 1

What do I crave? Bag of pretzels, coke

What can I do instead of eat? Go for a run

What could I eat instead of junk? Apple

Food actually eaten: Pretzels

Amount: ½ bag

Eventually you will see a change in your behavior. As you begin to realize how little your eating has to do with actual hunger, it will become easier to change the patterns. Most snacking is thoughtless, and just thinking about it will help you to control the forays into the refrigerator. Soon the run will replace the bag of pretzels. Let me know.

Most people who *have* to eat something *right this minute* are under the influence of the foraging center of the brain and low blood sugar. If you really feel hungry and nothing suggested above will distract you, the best thing to do is to eat six small meals a day. Save half of your lunch for the 3:00 P.M. slump. Nibble, nibble, nibble; but nibble on good foods—foods that only slowly release their calories.

How to Be a Healthier Snacker

Even if daily snacking remains a way of life for teens, there are steps you and your parents can take so that those extra snack calories are not all empty or fat-laden. A look at the food values of fast foods may inspire teens to arm themselves with their own snacks when they go off to the shopping malls with their friends after school or on weekends.

COMPOSITION OF FAST FOODS*

Item	Calories (g)	Protein (g)	Fats (g)	Carbo-hydrate (g)
Big Mac	541	26	31	39
Burger King Whopper	606	29	32	51
Burger Chef Hamburger	258	11	13	24
Dairy Queen Cheese Dog	330	15	19	24
Taco Bell Taco	186	15	8	14
Pizza Hut Thin 'N Crispy Cheese Pizza (½)	450	25	15	54
Pizza Hut Thick 'N Chewy Pepperoni Pizza (½)	560	31	18	68
Arthur Treacher's Fish Sandwich	440	16	24	39
Burger King Whaler	486	18	46	64
McDonald's Filet-o-Fish	402	15	23	34
Long John Silver's Fish (2 pieces)	318	19	19	19
Kentucky Fried Chicken Original Recipe Dinner	830	52	46	56
Kentucky Fried Chicken Extra Crispy Dinner (3 pieces)	950	52	54	63

* Jane Brody, *Jane Brody's Nutrition Book* (New York: Bantam Books, 1982), p. 397.

Item	Calories (g)	Protein (g)	Fats (g)	Carbo-hydrate (g)
McDonald's Egg McMuffin	352	18	20	26
Burger King French Fries	214	3	10	28
Dairy Queen Onion Rings	300	6	17	33
McDonald's Apple Pie	300	2	19	31
Burger King Vanilla Shake	332	11	11	50
McDonald's Chocolate Shake	364	11	9	60
Dairy Queen Banana Split	540	10	15	91

You can see that these fast food meals are much too high in calories and especially fats to serve as efficient snacks. And they don't compensate by being especially high in vitamins or minerals. Even as meals, most supply more than half of your daily caloric needs. The fried foods are especially high, as the frying often doubles the caloric value of the basic food.

When you add a soft drink to any of these you get about 150 added calories and 8 *teaspoons* of sugar. And the sodium content of most of these items is extremely high: 962 mg in a Big Mac, 836 mg in an Arthur Treacher's Fish Sandwich, 2,285 mg in a Kentucky Fried Chicken Original Recipe Dinner. The estimated safe and adequate daily dietary intake for sodium for people 11 years old and up is between 900 and 2,700 milligrams.

How Parents Can Help

- Replace sugary nothings and refined snacks with more nutritious equivalents (see the lists below and Martha

Rose's recipes), easily obtainable at natural foods stores and at many supermarkets. Keep these in opaque, covered containers. If you have bowls of snacks lying around, people will munch all day long.

- If you do have empty-calorie foods in the house, arrange cupboards and the refrigerator so that these foods aren't in sight, or are hard to reach. Out of sight, out of mind. Use your see-through containers for grains, beans, and wholegrain pasta.
- Always have cut-up vegetables, healthy dips, and fruit on hand, ready to eat.
- Use one refrigerator shelf just for snacks.
- Buy packaged foods in smaller bags.
- If you like to bake, use whole ingredients, such as whole wheat flour, cornmeal, oatmeal, honey, and sunflower seeds (see recipes).
- Save leftovers so your children can snack on the rest of their dinner, rather than sweets.

Techniques and Tricks

- Put away part of your dinner (like the dessert) and eat that when you get that yearning for an after-dinner snack.
- Snack on foods which are difficult to really overeat (because they are not empty foods). If you crave something really sweet, eat dried fruit, like figs. There are a lot of calories, but there is also a lot of food value there, and you will gag before you eat too much. Refined sugar is so refined that it gives you no warning when you've consumed too much. Use the lists below.
- Have the foods that you will snack on prepared in advance (vegetables cut up in plastic bags, wholesome cookies wrapped two to a packet, etc.), and try to snack at the same time every day.

- Always carry a supply of healthy food for eating in between meals. That way if you are with friends and snacking is what's on, you'll be armed with some food value.

- Try not to skimp on meals. If you eat well at meals, you won't be as tempted to snack. (Six smaller meals a day would keep your blood sugar even and hunger at a minimum.) Eat slowly and think about what you are eating. Enjoy each bite.

- If you can't resist eating ice cream or a chocolate-chip cookie, go ahead. But don't go overboard. Sometimes, because of the constant pressure to diet, once you "break down" and eat one cookie, you feel like you've lost some kind of battle, and you go ahead and eat another ten. Two cookies or a bowl of ice cream every once in a while are not going to kill you.

- Take your own popcorn and healthier candy to the movies.

- Use the soda pop ideas in this book to replace both regular *and* sugar-free soft drinks. Studies have shown that Nutrasweet, the sweetener used in diet sodas, can affect brain chemistry. It has been responsible for headaches, rashes, dizziness and menstrual problems.

Eat "comfort foods" that fill you up, not out. The foods that make the most popular snacks are comforting in some way. They are usually high in carbohydrates. So go for complex carbohydrates, rather than the empty refined kind. Snack on whole wheat pasta, granola, muffins, popcorn, whole grain bread, granola bars, homemade chips, the ice creams and ice pops suggested in this book, fruits, and vegetables. These are high in fiber and will fill you up before they do too much damage. See the section below for more recommendations. Make sure these foods are there and ready. If you are going to go to fast food places, look for salad bars and Mexican food, like burritos and bean tacos.

Foods for Snacking

Almost all of the foods that teens love to snack on can be replaced by healthier near-equivalents. Use these lists and recipes and trick yourselves into better snacking habits.

The following companies make candies, cookies, pastries, and snacks with reliable, whole ingredients such as whole wheat flour (vs. white flour), honey (vs. sugar), nuts, and grains.[1]

Arrowhead Mills	Health Valley
Barbara's Bakery	Lifestream
Better Way	Manna Mixins
Bronner	Natural Nectar
Caroba	Pure and Simple
Chico San	Schiff
De Boles	Shiloh Farms
De Sousa	Sonoma
Desert Gold	Sovex
Elf Liberty	Spicer's International
Erewhon	Stone Burr
Fearn	Walnut Acres
Hain	Westbrae

Candy

Suggested Products

Burry's and Caroba carob candies, chips, and carob-coated dried fruit and nuts

Naura Hayden's Dynamite Bar

Panda Licorice

Soken Plum Candy

Tania's Raisin-Nut Crunch, Sesame-Coconut Chews, Apricot-Cashew Crunch, and Maple-Nut Chews

Lifestream Sunshine Bar, Mega Bite, Hikers' Mix, Carob-Mint Fudge, Cashew Halvah, Sesame Dream

[1] For more information on trustworthy companies and alternative products, see Patricia McEntire, *Mommy, I'm Hungry* (Sacramento: Cougar Books, 1982), pp. 55–56, 88–91.

Natural Halvah: Carob, Cashew-Currant, and Plain

Chico San taffy and caramels

Golden Temple Wha Guru Chews: Original, Cashew-Almond, Sesame-Almond

Queen Bee Taffy

Nick's Treats

Burry's Carob Bars

Granola Bars

any of the dried fruit-and-nut mixes found in supermarkets and whole foods stores

Recipes

In the following recipes, the honey and molasses are only meant to be used once or twice, and then in decreasing amounts. As time goes by you will notice less of a need to have everything taste sweet. Experiment with fruit concentrates for the sweet flavor.

Mock Cracker Jacks

    4 cups popcorn
    1 cup dry roasted peanuts
    ½ cup sunflower seeds
    3 tablespoons margarine or safflower oil
    ¼ cup honey or maple syrup (approximately)

Preheat the oven to 350°. In a bowl, mix together all the ingredients except the honey; place on an oiled baking sheet. Roast in the oven for 15 to 20 minutes. Remove from the oven, return to the bowl, and stir in the honey or syrup (it will snap, crackle, and pop). Turn the oven down to 250°, place the mixture back on the baking sheet, and return to the oven. Bake another 10 to 15 minutes until the popcorn is golden. Remove, toss together well, and allow to cool.

Peanut Butter Candy

    ½ cup natural peanut butter
    ¼ cup honey (approximately—less is better; it can be done
      with none at all)

Up to ½ cup instant non-fat dry milk or ground sunflower seeds
Optional: ¼ cup raisins
        ¼ cup carob chips
        ¼ cup granola

Blend together the peanut butter and honey in an electric mixer or food processor. Add enough dry milk or ground sunflower seeds to make a stiff mixture with a doughlike consistency. Mix in the optional raisins, carob chips, or granola. Form into balls or log shapes and refrigerate on a covered plate or in plastic bags.

Dried Fruit and Nut Balls

¼ cup chopped walnuts
¼ cup sunflower seeds
¼ cup raisins
¼ cup chopped dried apricots
¼ cup rolled oats
¼ cup honey (approximately—just a smidge would be enough)
⅓ cup natural peanut butter

Combine the walnuts, sunflower seeds, raisins, dried apricots, and rolled oats. Stir in the honey and the peanut butter. Form into balls and refrigerate on a covered plate or in plastic bags.

Carob Peanut Butter Rounds

2 tablespoons honey (or use 2 teaspoons)
½ cup natural peanut butter
½ cup carob chips
¼ cup dried nonfat milk

Combine the honey and peanut butter, then mix in the carob chips and dried nonfat milk. Roll into a log shape and wrap in plastic wrap or wax paper. Chill several hours or place in the freezer for one hour. Cut into slices, wrap them individually, and keep in the refrigerator or freezer.

Peanut Butter Carob Fudge Balls

½ cup honey (approximately)   ¾ cup carob powder
1 cup natural peanut butter   ½ cup sunflower seeds

Mix together the honey and peanut butter and stir in the carob powder. Add the sunflower seeds. Roll into balls and refrigerate on a covered plate or in plastic bags.

Chocolate

Carob makes a wonderful substitute for chocolate. It is a powder ground from the pods of a tree and has a chocolatey flavor, with only half the fat, and lots of minerals and natural sugar.

See candy list, above, for suggested products.

Recipes

Hot Carob Syrup

    4 tablespoons butter
    4 tablespoons carob powder
¼–½ teaspoon nongranular instant decaffeinated coffee, to taste
    ¼ cup honey (you can get by with less or none)
    1 teaspoon vanilla

Melt the butter in a saucepan over low heat. Add the carob powder and coffee and mix together thoroughly with a wooden spoon. Stir in the honey and the vanilla and cook over low heat, stirring, for 5 minutes. This will become stiff when you cool it, and if you refrigerate it you could even substitute it for fudge.

Hot Carob Chocolate

    2 cups milk
    ¼ cup carob powder
    1 tablespoon honey (or less)

Blend together all the ingredients and heat to a simmer over medium heat.

Carob Brownies

    ½ cup safflower oil
    ⅔ cup honey (less is better; after a while you won't need any)
    2 eggs, beaten
    1 teaspoon vanilla extract

½ cup whole wheat pastry flour
¼ teaspoon salt
½ cup carob powder
½ cup sunflower seeds or broken walnuts

Preheat the oven to 350°; oil a 9-inch square baking pan or bread pan.

Cream together the oil and honey until the mixture is thick and creamy. Beat in the eggs and vanilla. Sift together the flour, carob powder, and salt. Stir into the liquid mixture and combine thoroughly. Stir in the sunflower seeds or walnuts.

Spread the batter in the oiled pan and bake for 25 to 35 minutes, until a tester comes out clean when inserted. Allow to cool in the pan until the sides of the brownie pull away from the pan, then reverse on a rack and cool completely. Cut into squares or slices and keep wrapped in foil.

Carob Molasses Brownies

Substitute 2 to 3 tablespoons blackstrap molasses (or more, as desired, but less, of course, is better) for the equivalent amount of honey and proceed as above.

Sodas

Health food stores now stock numerous brands of sodas made without sugar, colorings, or additives. There are also sparkling fruit juices, such as Martinelli's Sparkling Apple Cider, which easily fulfill the need for something bubbly and sweet.

Better still, and cheaper, make your own sodas, using one part fruit juice and one part club soda or sparkling mineral water, or two parts fruit juice and one part club soda or sparkling mineral water, to taste. See the recipes below.

Recipes

Fruit Soda 1

2 cups any fruit juice
1 cup club soda or sparkling mineral water (or use equal parts fruit juice and sparkling water)

Fruit Soda 2

1 cup orange juice
1 cup club soda or sparkling mineral water
1 cup cranberry juice

Fruit Soda 3

1 small can frozen fruit juice concentrate
1½ quarts club soda or sparkling mineral water

Dissolve the fruit juice concentrate in the club soda or sparkling mineral water and serve, or refrigerate in a sealed bottle.

Non–Ice Cream Soda

1 cup club soda
1 cup low-fat milk
2 tablespoons carob powder
1 teaspoon honey (or less)
2 teaspoons molasses (or less)
1 teaspoon vanilla
10 ice cubes

Blend together all the ingredients in a blender until the ice is thoroughly crushed, and serve.

Chips, Pretzels, and Savory Snacks

Suggested Products

Most whole foods stores now sell a variety of packaged foods that may still be high in fat, but at least they're made with whole-grain flours, unadulterated oils, and less salt. Health Valley, Soken, Bronners, Barbara's Bakery, Hain, Chico San, and Erewhon make chips and crackers such as:

cheese crackers
potato chips
pretzel twists and sticks
cheese puffs

  tortilla chips
  seaweed crackers
  multigrain crackers
  corn chips
  yogurt chips
  rice crackers
  puffed rice cakes
  Spicer Snacks
  Vege-Soy crackers

Other reliable products:

  Moo Munchies
  Tempura Chips
  Prothins
  Bran-a-Crisp
  Akmak Crackers

Recipes

Homemade Low-Fat Potato Chips

  1 potato, unpeeled and sliced very thin

Preheat the oven to 300°. Place the potato slices on a non-stick baking sheet. Bake for 40 minutes, or until thoroughly crisp and brown. You must watch them *very* carefully, because once they are thoroughly browned they will begin to burn right away. But if they aren't thoroughly browned they won't be crisp.

Homemade Low-fat Tortilla Chips

  12 corn tortillas, cut in wedges

Preheat the oven to 250°. Place the tortilla wedges on non-stick baking sheets and bake 40 minutes, or until crisp and beginning to brown.

Ice Cream

Both supermarkets and health food stores now stock ice pops made from fruit juice, with no extra sugar, and you can find ice cream made with fruit concentrate instead of sugar in health food stores. Frozen yogurt, Tofutti, and ice milk sweetened with fruit concentrates are better nutritional buys than regular ice cream. Natural Nectar makes great ice cream sandwiches, carob fudge bars, carob-coated vanilla bars, and ice cream or frozen yogurt between two granola cookies dipped in carob. Shiloh Farms makes honey ice cream, frozen yogurt, and ice pops. Many of these frozen treats are easy to make at home.

Recipes

See recipes for Banana Yogurt Ice Cream, Strawberry or Raspberry Ice, Frozen Apple Yogurt, Frozen Yogurt Popsicles, pp. 91, 92, 274, 275.

Frozen Fruit

Freeze bite-sized fruit, like grapes, strawberries, berries, and banana slices tossed in lemon juice or Vitamin C powder. These make fabulous low-calorie frozen treats. *For seedless grapes and berries:* Remove grapes from stems, freeze grapes and berries in plastic bags. *For bananas:* Slice and toss with lemon juice. Lay the slices on pieces of wax paper, cover with another sheet of wax paper, and freeze in a plastic bag.

Banana Ice Pops

Peel bananas and cut in half crosswise. Toss with lemon juice. Insert sticks and freeze in plastic bags.

Carob-Coated Banana Ice Pops

Peel bananas, cut in half crosswise, toss with lemon juice, and freeze as above. When frozen, dip in carob syrup and return to freezer.

Fruit Juice Ice Pops

Freeze fruit juice in ice pop molds (available at supermarkets and kitchen supply stores), or in paper cups. Cover the cups with foil and insert sticks in the middle. The foil holds up the stick.

Yogurt Ice Pops

Blend together plain low-fat yogurt and fresh fruit, such as berries or bananas, or try yogurt and fruit juice concentrate. Freeze in molds or paper cups, as above. Try the combinations below. Recipes serve 6.

Mixed Fruit and Yogurt Ice Pops

    1 pear or apple, chopped
    1 cup frozen or fresh strawberries
    ½ cup plain low-fat yogurt
    ½ cup orange juice, fresh or from concentrate
    ½ banana

Blend all the ingredients together until smooth and freeze in ice pop molds or paper cups.

Banana-Orange Yogurt Ice Pops

    1 cup plain low-fat yogurt (or substitute buttermilk)
    ½ cup orange juice, fresh or from concentrate
    1 banana

Blend together all the ingredients until smooth and freeze in ice pop molds or paper cups.

Strawberry Yogurt Ice Pops

    2 cups plain low-fat yogurt (or substitute buttermilk)
    1 cup orange juice from concentrate
    1 10-ounce package frozen strawberries
    2 tablespoons honey (or less, please)
    1 teaspoon vanilla (optional)

Blend together all the ingredients until smooth and freeze in ice pop molds or paper cups.

Pineapple Banana Mint Ice Pops

2 cups pineapple juice
1 banana
1 tablespoon fresh mint

Blend together all the ingredients until smooth and freeze in ice pop molds or paper cups.

Orange Yogurt Ice Pops

2 cups plain low-fat yogurt
1 tablespoon vanilla
1–2 tablespoons honey (teaspoon doses are better)
1 cup orange juice from concentrate

Blend together all the ingredients until smooth and freeze in ice pop molds or paper cups.

Carob Ice Pops

1 cup low-fat milk
1 cup plain low-fat yogurt
3 tablespoons carob powder
2 tablespoons honey (How about one to see how you're getting used to doing without?)
1 teaspoon vanilla
1 tablespoon molasses

Blend together all the ingredients and freeze in ice pop molds or paper cups.

Note: All the above frozen yogurt ice pop mixtures also make terrific smoothies for breakfast or snacks.

Pizza

If you're going to snack on fast food pizza, remove the cheese and sausage, and ask them not to douse with oil.

Many natural foods stores sell pizza with whole wheat

crusts. If they don't have whole pizzas, they almost all now stock
frozen whole wheat crusts, and several varieties of bottled tomato sauce. Armed with these ingredients you can put together
your own pizzas in no time. If you can't find any of these things,
try the recipes on page 254.

Your desire for pizza may be nothing more than a desire for
that wonderful taste of the bread and the Italian sauce. You can
satisfy this craving with whole wheat English muffins, pita, or
bread, spread with tomato sauce, sprinkled with a little low-fat
mozzarella or farmer's cheese and toasted under the broiler or in
a toaster oven. In fact, pizza can be one of the healthier snacks,
as long as you follow the above recommendations.

Fruit

Certainly fruit is one of the best items for snacking. Try to
vary your selection. If you are watching your calories, stick to no
more than four pieces a day.

Fruit Juice

Cut it with water or club soda to avoid getting the sugar so
quickly. Make sure no sugar is added. Frozen and filtered juices
are more sugar-concentrated than fresh unfiltered juices.

Carrots and Other Vegetables

Eat as many as you want. Try these other vegetables too.
They are the best snacks of all, because you can eat as much as
you want, and they can be eaten raw. Try to chew them 30 times
before swallowing. They should become like a soup in your
mouth.

asparagus
green beans
beets
broccoli
cabbage
cauliflower

celery
cucumbers
endive
escarole
lettuce of all kinds
mushrooms
red or green peppers
tomatoes
zucchini

Pep them up with the following dips:

plain mustard
vinegar
lemon juice
soy sauce
any of the Low-Fat Vinaigrettes on pages 219 and 220
Salsa Fresca (page 258)
low-fat yogurt with added herbs or spices
natural peanut butter
cottage cheese with chives
low-fat yogurt with a health food soup mix
Hummus (see page 217)

Tahini Dip 1

½ cup sesame tahini
juice of 1 lemon
  1 clove garlic

Tahini Dip 2

  ½ cup sesame tahini
1–2 tablespoons soy sauce
  1 teaspoon freshly grated ginger (or ¼–½ teaspoon
    powdered)

Spinach Yogurt Dip

10 ounces frozen spinach, thawed
juice of ½ lemon
¼–½ cup plain low-fat yogurt (to taste)

Blend together the above ingredients in a food processor or blender until smooth.

Toast

Use whole-grain breads and replace butter with natural peanut butter, sesame tahini, unsweetened fruit preserves, or health margarine.

Chinese Food

Avoid fried foods, like egg rolls, and high fat meats, like spare ribs, beef, and pork. Chinese food is usually a meal in itself, so save it for lunch or dinner if you really have a craving for it, and snack on something else. When you do order it, go for vegetables, tofu, seafood, or chicken dishes.

Peanut Butter and Jelly Sandwich

Use natural peanut butter, with no added oil, sugar, or salt, and whole-grain bread. Replace sugary jellies with unsweetened fruit preserves, now available in natural foods stores, or mashed bananas. (Wax Orchards in Vashon Island, Washington, has great fruit spreads, all natural.)

Chocolate Milk

Substitute carob powder for chocolate and use skim milk or soy milk. For each cup of milk blend in 1 tablespoon carob powder, ½ teaspoon honey, and ½ teaspoon vanilla.

Chicken

Remove the skin. Avoid fast food fried chicken. See the chart on pages 79–80 for the calorie statistics.

Nuts

Eat raw or dry-roasted nuts. Avoid salty nuts which have been roasted in oil.

Cookies and Pastries

See the companies listed in the beginning of this section. Most of the companies that make healthy candies and snacks also make baked goods. Many natural foods stores have their own bakeries and sell wholesome cookies and pastries by the piece, precisely because people like to munch while they're shopping.

If pastries are your weakness, go for fruit pies instead of cakes. At least you'll be getting some fruit, and the pies have less butter and sugar than other pastries. Better still, try the *muffins* on pages 198–203.

Recipes

Peanut Butter Banana Cookies

¼ cup safflower oil
½ cup mild-flavored honey (try to get by with less)
 2 eggs
½ teaspoon vanilla extract
½ cup peanut butter
 1 cup mashed, ripe banana
¾ cup whole wheat pastry flour
 1 teaspoon double-acting baking powder
¼ teaspoon salt

Preheat the oven to 350°. Lightly oil nonstick baking sheets.
Cream together the oil and the honey. Beat in the eggs, peanut butter, and mashed banana. Sift together the flour, baking powder, and salt, and stir into the liquid mixture. Blend well.

Drop onto prepared baking sheets by scant tablespoonfuls and bake 12 to 15 minutes. Cool on racks. (Makes 4 dozen cookies.)

Oatmeal Carob Chip Cookies

    1 cup raisins
Boiling water to cover
1 ½ cups sifted whole wheat pastry flour
    ¼ teaspoon salt
    ½ teaspoon baking soda
    1 teaspoon cinnamon
    ½ teaspoon nutmeg
    ½ teaspoon allspice
    ½ cup safflower margarine (available at health food stores)
    ½ cup mild-flavored honey (less is better)
    1 teaspoon vanilla extract
    2 eggs
    2 cups rolled or flaked oats
    1 cup carob chips

Place the raisins in a saucepan or bowl and pour on boiling water to cover. Let stand 5 to 10 minutes, then drain, reserving ⅓ cup of the water. Pat the raisins dry between sheets of paper towel.

Preheat the oven to 350°. Lightly oil nonstick baking sheets.

Sift together the flour, salt, baking soda, and spices, and set aside.

Cream the margarine and add the honey. Beat well. Beat in the vanilla, then the eggs, one at a time. Slowly beat in the oats, then the raisins, beating just to mix. Beat in the water reserved from the raisins, then slowly add the sifted dry ingredients, scraping the bowl and beating only until mixed. Stir in the carob chips.

Drop by large teaspoonfuls onto lightly oiled nonstick baking sheets, about 2 inches apart. Bake 12 to 15 minutes, reversing the sheets halfway through the baking, until the cookies are golden brown and the tops spring back when lightly pressed with a fingertip. Cool on racks. (Makes 4 dozen cookies.)

Carob Raisin Cookies

    4 ounces carob chips
    2 cups sifted whole wheat pastry flour
    ¼ cup sifted soy flour

½ teaspoon baking soda
¼ teaspoon salt
½ cup safflower margarine or oil
½ cup mild-flavored honey (when you try it again, skip the
    honey—the raisins should make it sweet enough)
2 tablespoons molasses
1 teaspoon vanilla extract
1 egg
½ cup plain yogurt
1 cup raisins

Preheat the oven to 375°. Lightly oil nonstick baking sheets.

Melt the carob chips in the top part of a double boiler over boiling water.

Sift together the flours, baking soda, and salt, and set aside. Cream the margarine or oil with the honey, molasses and vanilla. Beat in the egg, then the melted carob and the yogurt. Gradually add the dry ingredients, beating at low speed and scraping the sides of the bowl with a rubber spatula, only until the ingredients are blended together. Stir in the raisins.

Drop by heaping teaspoons onto the baking sheets, about 2 inches apart. Bake 15 to 20 minutes in the preheated oven, reversing the sheets top to bottom and front to back halfway through to insure even baking. The cookies are done when they spring back lightly when pressed with fingertips. Remove from the oven and cool on racks. (Makes 5 dozen cookies.)

Carob Chip Cookies

½ cup safflower margarine
⅔ cup mild-flavored honey (less is okay, too)
2 eggs
1 teaspoon vanilla
2 cups sifted whole wheat pastry flour
½ teaspoon baking soda
¼ teaspoon salt
½ cup chopped walnuts or sunflower seeds
1 cup carob chips

Preheat the oven to 375°. Lightly oil nonstick baking pans.

Cream together the margarine and honey. Beat in the eggs and vanilla. Sift together flour, baking soda, and salt. Stir into the wet ingredients. Stir in the carob chips and nuts or sunflower seeds.

Drop by heaping teaspoons onto the baking sheets and bake 12 minutes in the preheated oven. Cool on racks. (Makes 5 dozen cookies.)

Carrot Cake

¾ cup safflower oil
½ cup honey (try to use less)
1 tablespoon molasses
4 eggs
1 teaspoon vanilla extract
1 cup sifted whole wheat flour
¼ cup sifted soy flour
1 cup unbleached white flour
1 ½ teaspoons baking powder
1 ½ teaspoons cinnamon
1 ½ teaspoons nutmeg
½ teaspoon salt
½ pound carrots, grated
1 cup raisins

Preheat the oven to 350°. Butter a large loaf pan or Bundt pan.

Cream the oil with the honey and molasses until the mixture is fluffy. Beat in the eggs and vanilla.

Sift together the flours, baking powder, spices, and salt. Stir into the liquid ingredients and beat until the mixture is smooth, then stir in the grated carrots and the raisins.

Pour the batter into the pan and bake in the preheated oven for one hour, until a toothpick inserted in the center comes out clean.

Let cool in the pan until it pulls away from the sides, then reverse onto a rack. Cool and slice thinly.

Popcorn

Pop your own in a dry popper, or using a small amount of safflower oil. Instead of tossing with butter and salt, try other seasonings, like curry, dry mustard, paprika, kelp, cumin. Popcorn is one of the easiest low-calorie snacks.

Burritos

See recipe, page 251. If you are eating in a restaurant or fast food place, ask them to omit the cheese. Many natural foods stores now carry delicious packaged burritos.

Fries

Avoid. Sorry, but there's no way to make a low-fat French fry.

Bagels

Buy whole wheat, rye, or pumpernickel bagels. Substitute Low-Fat "Cream Cheese," page 205, for real cream cheese. A good way to enjoy bagels is to scoop out the bread, throw it away, and toast the crust in the oven. Fill with low-fat cottage cheese for a delicious, healthy treat.

Burgers

Avoid eating hamburgers between meals, because they already supply about one-third to one-half your daily calorie requirements. Try to find whole wheat buns and don't pour on lots of ketchup, which is full of sugar.

Tofu and bean burgers are now easy to find in health food stores and snack bars.

Cereal

Choose from the approved list of cereals on page 154. Moisten with skim milk. Sweeten with fruit or a little honey.

Remember, it's never too early—or too late—to start feeding yourself right.

CHAPTER 5

The Doctor-Teenager Relationship: Happiness in the Doctor's Office

During the adolescent years not only do relationships between children and their parents change, but relationships between teenagers and their doctors also change. Sensitivity on the part of the pediatrician or the family physician is most important during this time. The child he once treated for chicken pox may now come to him with problems which might be embarrassing—most are, at least, intimate. The teenager needs to feel that he can confide in his doctor, and that, even though the doctor may have known him since he was in diapers, Dr. X doesn't have the same kind of expectations that his parents do.

TO THE TEENAGER: You have worked around the childhood tilts and torques; you are getting to an age where you can almost always get what you want from your parents, and you are having some fun. You have even made a few friends. Now what? You are struck with puberty. Talk about stress!

You start to talk back to your parents, as they suddenly seem to want to run your life. The word "rebellion" crops up; *you* thought it was just more rapid growth and development. You make phone calls and have meetings with friends to discuss personal things; you need friends. You need intimacy, but with a same-sex chum, not your parents. They really seem old-fashioned. You love them, but they are too removed from what's happening.

You grow a couple of inches a year. You are tired if you have chores, but have energy if a friend calls and wants to do something fun. Your parents do not understand all this, so you are taken to the pediatrician or family doctor who has known you all your life. Mononucleosis and anemia are ruled out.

"Is he (she) sick? If nothing's wrong, we may have to apply a little pressure," your folks say.

"He's (she's) normal. Just an adolescent."

What a relief, you think. (He: But why is my penis so small? She: Why is one breast larger than the other?) But how do you really know if you're normal?

TO THE PARENTS: I found that after the exam and history-taking with the budding pubescent and the parent present, I would ask the mother or father to leave the room so I could ask the youth some questions in private. How is school and life in general? Most would say, "It's okay."

"Are you concerned about your organs?"

"A little."

"Do you want to talk about it?"

"Not especially."

"Here's my number. Why don't you call me some day?"

Few did. Years later some of their parents told me that their child kept that phone number in a safe place in the desk at home. I had become a part of the extended family. I was also learning to be accepting of a wide variety of lifestyles. I had to— partly because it was good for business, but mainly, I hope, it was because these were human beings groping for some answers, and I was part of the process.

Something else I learned: pubescent young people should not be pushed into dating or sexual relations until they find they are ready. They are searching for their identity during those early adolescent years. They need to share feelings and thoughts with a chum, but there is a loneliness until they know who they are. They are looking for their "way of life," testing the environment. They are action-oriented; some are impulsive, some aggressive, and some sexual.

The mid-adolescent (girls 12 to 15 years old, boys 14 to 17) needs to experiment with different identities, but on safe ground and with plenty of escape mechanisms available. "No, I can't; my folks would kill me." "If they find out, I'm grounded for a week." Parents need to provide rules. Many adolescents feel more secure with the rules although they complain about rigidity and the archaic style of their parents.

TO THE TEENAGER: Your doctor should provide an atmosphere of comfort, trust, respect, and confidence so that you may talk freely about sexual activity, anxieties, depression, and drug use. The doctor may not know what to *do* about what you are telling him, but just *talking* about sensitive issues may be enough to suggest a method of handling them. Everyone is different. You may do better with a doctor of the same sex. If you feel you need to change doctors for this reason, your present doctor should understand.

When establishing a relationship with a physician, the minimal requirements should be that he or she is well-informed, uses simple language, and, most important, has a *nonjudgmental attitude.*[1] You and your doctor should be assured of privacy (a chance to talk without your parents).

Let us assume that you are having a physical examination at the doctor's office. The doctor should at least ask, "How're you doing?" It is a nice open-ended question to get the conversation going. You should be honest with your doctor; you would like to respond:

"I get nervous and my palms sweat and my heart races. Some nights I cannot sleep and I have occasional headaches, stomachaches, and a backache after I exercise. I get down in the dumps every once in a while and wonder 'What's the point?' and throw my books in the corner and cry. My Mom says it's a phase, but I don't know. I get real tired in school after lunch; the

[1] Susan M. Coupey, M.D., "Medical Interviews with Adolescents," *Medical Aspects of Human Sexuality,* vol. 18, Dec. 12, 1984, pp. 65–70.

teacher keeps the room too hot. I'm fat. How can I lose ten pounds by next week?"

But it seems safer to tell the doctor: "Mom says I have a wart on my foot; can you put some stuff on it? And do you have some antihistamine samples for my hay fever? The pills I use now put me to sleep."

The doctor is delighted that you have asked him to do something for you; doctors want to be helpful with specific complaints. That may have been the best thing you could have done for yourself and the doctor; you allowed him to be comfortable with you. He refers you to a dermatologist for the plantar wart and gives you a handful of samples from the drawer.

Now is the time to tell him your real complaints. He is in the mood for listening as you have helped the doctor establish the "doctor-patient relationship." (If you are surly and noncommunicative, sitting with a curled lip and folded arms, you tell the doctor you don't like him or his advice. It is best to play the doctor game in his office. Be cheerful and compliant—doctors like that. Some day you may want him to treat you for some nasty, painful disease.) So you tell him of your concerns and he is sympathetic. He nods and says, "I see," but he feels your symptoms are *average*; because he hears this litany of complaints from so many of his patients, he assumes they are *normal*. But normality is freedom from pain and anxiety accompanied by an exuberance of life. However, if you are naked on the cold examining table with some paper sheets between you and the world, your lack of comfort may be so distracting that when the doctor asks more about your symptoms, all you can respond with is, "I'm okay, I guess."

There is no way the doctor can live inside your body and understand your perception of your world. But the above-average doctor, the kind you should look for, although he has no way of actually measuring your feelings, should be sympathetic and imaginative enough to understand them. Many doctors assume that if you are warm, your blood pressure is okay, your tonsils are not enlarged, and your blood tests are within the normal limits, if there is no pus in your urine and he can find no muscle spasm, no bloat nor lump, then you are "normal" and any subjective complaints mean you have a tranquilizer deficiency or you need the shrink. Even if you tell the average doctor you are depressed or anxious or you cannot sleep, he only knows that there is a drug for every condition. He is a medical doctor, for heaven's sake.

He may also be filing your complaints next to the memories of his own complaints and problems when he was your age, and knows that *he* somehow survived. He might agree with your mother's diagnosis: "It's a phase."

In the August 1984 issue of the journal *Pediatrics* (page 196), in the summary of an article about adolescents, "Resident Skills in Adolescent Care,"[2] the author states: "Pediatric and medical residents appear to have important deficiencies in their training with regard to the care of adolescent patients." And these M.D.s are but a few months away from starting their own private practices. Apparently some of them have forgotten how they felt when they were 12 to 18 years of age; or if they remember how they felt, it is too traumatic a memory to relive it with every adolescent that comes through the office door.

We expect the doctor to be knowledgeable about medical things; he learned how to make diagnoses in his training. But the ability to be sympathetic was learned at home, from his or her parents. If you feel that your doctor is not sympathetic, shop around for a new one. Adolescence is a normal time to change doctors. You can't choose your parents, but you can choose your physician. And if you're not happy with a medical doctor's responses to what you feel may be problems with nutritional causes, try a visit to a licensed nutritionist or naturopath. You are going through a stressful time and need all the support systems available.

[2] Gail Slap, M.D., M.S., "Adolescent Medicine," *Pediatrics*, vol. 74, August 1984, pp. 191–197.

CHAPTER 6

The Best Way to Eat

Modern-day scientific and processing advances have made food more available and possibly cheaper, but the human intestinal tract has not changed from what it was when our ancestors ate raw foods. It is still waiting for the food it was designed to digest.

Certain digestive enzymes are necessary to digest and absorb the foods we swallow and they in turn require certain vitamins and minerals to function optimally. Somehow God and Mother Nature figured this all out and put the required amounts of vitamins and minerals into the foods we are supposed to eat. But food processing and soil depletion, cooking and storage have reduced these ingredients to a level that makes human digestion difficult. You have seen the ads for most commercial cereals. The manufacturers cheerfully indicate how thoughtful and generous they are because they have added 9 vitamins and minerals. Big deal. They forgot to mention that they removed 29 important vitamins and minerals during the processing. The commercial dessert cupcakes many of you pack in your lunches are so "pure" (pure sugar and refined flour and hydrogenated fat) they will last years on the shelf.

The rule is: Eat foods that *can* rot, but eat them before they *do* rot.

Did you ever wonder why you prefer to eat fruits that have just ripened? They are sweet, that's why. And the taste is connected with the pleasure center of the brain. I would propose that we are encouraged to eat sweet fruit because Mother Nature wants us to eat the fruit when the vitamin C is most abundant.

If we would imitate our distant relatives who followed animal migrations millions of years ago, we would be eating meat and vegetables. Paleontologists tell us, however, that the meat they ate was very low in fat—just under 4 percent. Remember, those were wild animals our ancestors were chasing. They were lean. The animals we eat today are steers and pigs who have been standing around in feedlots staring into space. Many of them are still getting hormones to increase the fat content of the meat, which is 30 percent after the visible fat has been removed!

I don't know how they figured it out, but the type of fat our ancestors ate was high in omega-3 fats (gamma linoleic and linolenic) which tend to encourage the production of prostaglandin E-1, an anti-inflammatory substance. Meat eaters today get arachidonic acid, which leads to prostaglandin E-2, an inflammatory substance. Nathan Pritikin, an advocate of a low-fat, low-sugar diet, was able to clear his own and most of his clients' blood vessels of atherosclerotic sludge because he followed a regimen of exercise and a low-fat, mostly vegetable diet. It works. Our bodies were not designed to eat modern "food."

We need calories, and adolescents usually need a *lot* of calories for growth and energy. All the nutritional research indicates that we do better if we eat as little fat and sugar as possible. Most of us do better if we get our vitamins, minerals, energy, and roughage from vegetable sources.

What about fruit? It is a little better than sugar out of the sugar bowl. Research has found that if fruits (or sugar) are eaten with protein, the body's ability to digest the protein is impaired. Bacterial action putrefies the protein and the victim has a lot of smelly gas. Bad on a date. Eat it alone or leave it alone.

The Mini-Meal Method

Try eating mini-meals four to six times a day. These meals should feature small amounts of low-fat protein like fish or turkey or chicken (without the skin)—just one ounce at a time. Or use lentil or bean soup for your protein, along with some whole grains like a piece of whole wheat or rye bread. The mini-meal should also feature vegetables and complex carbohydrates—but eat the protein first, so that plenty of stomach acid will be available for the breakdown of protein.

Protein

All meat contains protein but not all protein is contained in meat. Protein consists of amino acids—chains of carbon atoms plus hydrogen, at least one nitrogen atom, and some oxygen atoms. Some have a sulfur atom. (Rotten eggs give off hydrogen sulfide.) The liver can make some of the amino acids we need daily from other amino acids, but some—called essential amino acids—need to be consumed daily to provide for the repair of tissue, to aid in the production of the immune system cells and globulins, and to form parts of the enzymes.

Until recently it was thought that if you ate some meat and drank some milk every day, you were bound to get all the amino acids you needed (essential and nonessential), along with some extra just in case. But now that we have gotten used to that rather high protein intake, it has been determined that the fat content of these foods is too much for the health of our blood vessels, and for our attempts to stay slim.

Vegetarians have known this for decades and are demonstrating that they are on the right pathway to health. They have fewer degenerative diseases (less high blood pressure, osteoporosis, obesity, diabetes, arthritis, and constipation). However, they sometimes suffer from anemia and low protein (albumin) levels in the blood.

With a minimum of thinking ahead most of us can get enough of the essential and nonessential amino acids through the consumption of vegetables alone, thus avoiding the potential hazards of the high amount of fat accompanying the present-day animal protein. (The new beefalo is supposed to be low in fat, and tastes almost like beef.)

Of course, during periods of rapid growth and great metabolic demands, an increased intake of protein is necessary. One

such period occurs in the first days of infancy: if a baby continued to grow at the same rate as in the first two weeks of life, by
the time 10 years had gone by, he would be 22 feet tall. Another
growth spurt hits adolescents; they seem to grow before our very
eyes! Four inches a year is a strain. The intestines do not absorb
every calorie swallowed, so the youth must eat huge amounts to
avoid the pain and tension of hunger. About 1 gram of protein is
needed for each kilogram (2.2 pounds) of weight per day to
accommodate for the losses and supply the needs of the growing
tissues. That translates to about 70 grams (2 ounces) of good-
quality protein for a 150-pound person.

No piece of food is all protein; food tables tell us of the
relative percentages of protein in the different foods. A quarter
of a pound of most fish has about 20 grams of protein. An egg
has 6 grams of protein. A cup of cottage cheese has 30 grams of
protein. But a cup of cooked oatmeal has about 5 grams of protein, and the same number of grams of protein is in a cup of
enriched spaghetti and most pasta. A cup of split-pea soup has 8
or 9 grams of protein. So you can do pretty well with fish and
vegetable and grain and dairy sources of protein and be less
dependent upon high-fat, expensive red meat.

High-Protein Foods

LOW-FAT FISH

Food	Quantity	Protein (g)
Bass	¼ pound	21
Cod	¼ pound	20
Flounder, sole	¼ pound	19
Halibut	¼ pound	23
Snapper	¼ pound	22
Swordfish	¼ pound	22
Tuna, canned in water	1 cup	56
Oysters	¼ pound	9
Scallops	¼ pound	17
Salmon, fresh	¼ pound	25

LOW-FAT FOWL AND GAME

Food	Quantity	Protein (g)
Turkey	¼ pound	34
Chicken breast	¼ pound	20
Venison	¼ pound	24

LOW-FAT VEGETABLES

Food	Quantity	Protein (g)
Alfalfa sprouts, raw	1 cup	5
Black-eyed peas, cooked	1 cup	13
Lentils, cooked	1 cup	15
Lima beans, cooked	1 cup	15
Red kidney beans, cooked	1 cup	14
Soybean curd (tofu)	3 ounces	8

Most cheeses have the same amount of fat as protein. They are now called fatty foods.

LOW-FAT DAIRY PRODUCTS

Food	Quantity	Protein (g)
Cottage cheese	1 cup	30
Mozzarella, part skim	1 ounce	8
Parmesan, hard	1 ounce	10
Buttermilk	1 cup	8

HIGH-FAT MEAT

Food	Quantity	Protein (g)
Ground beef, regular	¼ pound	20
T-bone steak	¼ pound	116
Lamb chops	¼ pound	16
Bacon, sliced	¼ pound	9

Sausage and luncheon meats are about as bad as bacon. Veal has a little less fat than protein per weight.

HIGH-CHOLESTEROL, LOW-FAT SEAFOOD

Food	Quantity	Protein (g)
Clams	4 large ones	14
Crabs, steamed	¼ pound	20
Lobster	¼ pound	19

Energy Foods: Complex Carbohydrates

The wisest plan is to get calories for energy from fruits, vegetables, and cereal foods, and use the protein foods mainly for tissue growth, metabolic needs, and the immune system.

Because protein can be converted to energy, it was thought just a few years ago that a high-protein diet would be the best way to control the weakness, mental confusion, and irritability of hypoglycemia. The hypoglycemic was to eat two eggs for breakfast, have a chicken leg at 10:00 A.M., tuna salad at noon, a chunk of cheese at 3:00 P.M., a steak for dinner, and nuts and seeds at appropriate intervals in between. It did work, but the high-protein diet was expensive, had too much fat, and was a load on the liver. Our distant ancestors, at least, were able to feast on low-fat animals. It was soon discovered that these hypoglycemic folks did better if they stayed away from the sweets and the fats, and tried to get their energy from complex carbohydrates.

Complex carbohydrates are our best source of energy because they are broken down into usable sugar at such a slow rate that they are less likely to stimulate the flow of insulin which tends to make us crave food. Starchy foods have energy, of course, but they require the saliva (chew them 30 times before swallowing) and an enzyme from the pancreas, amylase, to break them down to simple carbohydrates before they can be absorbed. (Simple sugars are easily digested and are absorbed rapidly.)

Among the complex carbohydrates are most vegetables, especially corn, squash, potatoes, and similar foods. Whole-grain foods are good forms of complex carbohydrates. But white bread, cake, and refined-flour pasta do not provide enough roughage, fiber, B vitamins, and minerals to allow them to be metabolized effectively.

Always ask for whole-grain bread. Try to use whole-grain pasta. Brown rice or wild rice is better than white rice. Try to get energy and sustenance from vegetables, as we need the vitamins and minerals from these foods to allow our digestive enzymes to work.

Vegetables

The vegetables provide some vitamins, some minerals, and energy. These bonuses are wrapped up in the cells which our digestive juices have to break down before we can use the glucose from the starches. This gives us the long, slow, even energy that is the best for our bodies.

Vegetables are best eaten raw, or steamed, or cooked using the quick-fry method in the wok. One should chew, chew, chew vegetables until they are but a soup in the mouth, then swallow. This salivary digestion is important to start the digestion of the complex carbohydrates, the starches.

In any given meal or snack, the roots, like potatoes, carrots, beets, turnips, and rutabagas, should be eaten first; then the white vegetables like cauliflower and onions; then the green ones like Brussels sprouts, asparagus, and broccoli; and then the purple cabbage. The quick energy from sugar is too quickly dissipated and most of us are left on the floor or with a migraine.

Eat the salad last. Lettuce, endive, spinach leaves—the green leafy vegetables—should be eaten last of all. If you are in a restaurant, and they serve the salad first to shut you up, tell them that you are French and you want the entree first and the salad last. You should have the protein first to take advantage of the higher concentration of stomach acid.

Snacks

In between these mini-meals you may have some fruit and nuts and seeds. I do best with an apple and 16 almonds. It seems to hold me until the next "meal" of a cold piece of turkey and some raw or steamed broccoli.

This is the stone-age diet: Avoid dairy products, eat fruits in season, concentrate on vegetables, and toss down a little protein or some meat you have chased and brought down yourself. Try to imitate the ways of your ancient ancestors. You cannot run naked through the woods eating bark, leaves, berries, and small rodents that might get in your way, but you can concentrate on the veggies, fruits, nuts, and whole grains. You probably will still eat greasy hamburgers, sugared cereals, fat-laden cheese, and soft drinks with sugar, but you don't have to eat them all the time. Compromise, compromise. Be slow and gradual, but see if, after a month, some of your chronic symptoms go away.

I was taught—as you must have been—that there are four basic food groups: fruits and vegetables, grains (bread and cereal), protein (meat, eggs, and fish), and the dairy products. It is an easy way to remember all the edible things on the earth, and the balance seems to be pretty good, but it may come as no surprise to you to learn that this was put together by the American Dairy Council. It was not based on any scientific investigation, except perhaps the observation that cows produced more milk than their calves needed, and that if the farmers continued to milk the cows, the cows continued to give milk. We are using this food in a way that Mother Nature did not intend. (Similarly, the egg was meant to make a chicken, not to feed us.)

Researchers in cardiovascular disease suggest new food groups for optimal health.

The main group is *vegetables,* as little cooked as possible.

Next in importance are the *lean meats,* especially fish, chicken (without the skin), and occasional eggs. The deep-sea, cold-water fish are the ones to concentrate on, as they are more likely to have the omega-3 fats. Lean meats would be used as condiments to the vegetables

On a roughly equal standing with the meats are *whole grains (cereals and breads) and legumes (beans):* these, combined with one another, provide complete proteins, as they offer all the essential amino acids needed for growth, tissue repair, and immune-system strength.

Next is a group of foods to be eaten only when seasonally available: *nuts, seeds, and fruit.*

The *low-fat dairy products* should be eaten only occasionally: yogurt, skim milk, low-fat cheese.

And on the bottom of the list are *recreational foods,* which should be taken only if a friend forces you to eat them at a party: fat, sugar, salt, and white, bleached flour. Try to eat some good, nutritious food before you get into the ding-dongs.

Most of us have found that if we eat the foods recommended above—small amounts frequently—we feel better, we maintain a normal weight, and have normal bowel movements once or twice a day.

Obviously we are all different, and what works on one may not work on another. What foods you have been reared on will largely determine what you will tend to eat now. My mother used to say, "You cannot ruin good food." She could. My wife makes mediocre food taste delicious. I finish my plate no matter how much is on it because my mother locked the idea into my brain. So with good-tasting food (sugary and fatty) on the plate, it is hard to stay trim.

It is not too late to change some habits. See if your diet is following along the lines of the present recommendations: 20 percent or less of calories should come from fat (remember Pritikin was down to 10 percent fat and had clean blood vessels), 15 percent from protein, and the rest from complex carbohydrates.

CHAPTER 7

Five Diet Plans for Teenagers

To Teenagers and Their Parents

One fact needs to be reemphasized: We are all different. We all have different nutritional needs. Our thoughts, feelings, and perceptions are based on genetic factors and past experiences, but we all have the need to feel good about ourselves and our world. Without food that has sustaining potential, we would be weak and discouraged. Without food that has the required minerals and vitamins and roughage, the enzymes that turn swallowed food into useful nutriments for brain and body cannot work.

To Teenagers:

The following diet plans will all allow for normal body and brain function. They have enough protein, fiber, complex carbohydrates, and a smidge of fat. They are easy to fix. I hate to say this, but they are good for you, or anyone!

Almost everyone thinks better and feels more energetic if their three meals are split into six mini-meals. As Martha Rose suggests, the habit of nibbling on raw vegetables is the best way to sustain the blood sugar between the meals. I know many teenagers who refuse to eat breakfast and seem to do okay. That is their style. But if you think that eating but one meal a day is the way to lose weight, you are mistaken.

(I wonder if your disinterest in eating with your parents in the morning is based more on the negative comments you know you will hear when they see your clothes or your hairstyle. You may be dying of hunger, but you don't need to be criticized for your perception of the appropriate thing to wear so early in the day. Many parents don't hesitate to berate their sons and daughters at breakfast; a quick way for everyone to lose their appetite.)

To the Parents:

Assume that a part of your inability to feed your teenager properly is based on the natural rebellion of the age group; allow for choices and an occasional retreat into the apparently bottomless and endlessly appealing abyss of the junk food world. The diets in this book are all good and have all the right things in them. If you cannot get your teen to accept these as a way of life, at least *aim* for this ideal. When your son or daughter is twenty-five years old, he or she will probably ask you why you didn't make him or her eat better as a youngster. You'll respond, "Heaven knows I tried."

The usual rebuttal will be: "You didn't try hard enough."

Some people are nauseated in the morning because they are in acidosis from eating something sugary-sweet the night before. To shove food down a reluctant throat is inviting an emetic return. The parent who accepts this and is willing to compromise can at least put some raw almonds or walnuts and an apple in the teen's (or spouse's) jacket pocket and hope that this healthy snack will be discovered before the blood sugar drops so low that brain function slips to the animal, spinal cord level.

A man told me that, as a boy in the thirties when he came home from school in the afternoon, he first went into the backyard garden and pulled up a root vegetable—turnip, parsnip, carrot, radish, or whatever, wiped the dirt off on his pants, and ate it fresh. He, of course, got calories, vitamins, minerals, fiber, and energy and alertness. It was cheap, too. (Think how we are getting cheated financially and nutritionally when we eat the potato chips instead of the potato.) Try to imitate how our ancestors ate; we still have the same intestinal tract they did. Our gut was made to eat foods in their natural, unprocessed state.

To the Teenager:

Okay, so you have gotten this far in the book and are motivated to *do* something about:

1. flabby bulges. If you can see or feel the fat deposits, you are to remember that the muscles have run out of storage places, and this bulge represents the overflow.

2. the long wait to get good food. You find you do better if you eat frequently, but you cannot start up your Coleman stove in the middle of the school parking lot, or in team practice, or on the walk or ride home.

3. the greasy pimples. You know that food is 50 percent of the trouble but you don't know where to start. You don't want to take antibiotics because you have heard how they can muck up your immune system. The diet approach to a good complexion is rewarding but it is slow.

4. food sensitivities. About 60 percent of us are sensitive to foods, wheat and milk being the top two. (Close behind: corn, soy, and eggs.) Sensitivities can give gas, nausea, diarrhea, headaches, rashes, surliness, and depression.

5. being underweight. You are a girl and realize that you are really scrawny; you think no boy would want to grab you. You are a boy and want to build up a little muscle mass so you will look a little more mature. (This will only work, however, if you have some curly pubic hair, which is a sign that you have testosterone, and your muscles will then respond to exercise and diet.)

Here are five diet plans designed to meet the multiple needs of teenagers. Each plan consists of three breakfast, lunch, and dinner choices, as well as snack suggestions. Recipes for dishes marked with an asterisk (*) can be found in Chapter 11. For an all-around family plan, see Chapter 11.

It is important with all these diets to try, as much as possible, without wasting food, to rotate the foods you eat. Try not to have dairy products, or wheat foods, or corn or eggs, and even soy beans, more than once every four days or so. These foods are more likely to be allergenic and even produce some startling cravings and addictions in some people who are so predisposed.

Diet 1: Quickest Weight-Loss Diet

This is a very low-calorie diet, with few natural sugars and fewer, though sufficient, complex carbohydrates than the other diets. There are also very few desserts. If you feel hungry on this diet, eat as many raw vegetables in between meals as you like. You may season them with mustard, lemon juice, or vinegar.

BREAKFAST   1 cup nonfat plain yogurt
             ½ grapefruit
             Herb tea, unsweetened

LUNCH   1 cup Gazpacho* with 2 ounces cubed tofu, tossed
             with soy sauce
             Crudités*
             1 apple, pear, or orange
             Water (can be sparkling mineral water or club soda)

DINNER   Fish Teriyaki* (3½-ounce serving, or Poached Filet
             of Sole with Tomato Puree*
             ⅓ cup brown rice
             Steamed spinach or broccoli
             Tossed green salad with Low-Fat Vinaigrette*
             Water

BREAKFAST   1 soft-boiled egg
             1 slice whole wheat toast (dry)
             6 ounces fresh orange juice
             Herb tea, unsweetened

LUNCH   ½ cup Tuna Salad*
             Crudités*
             1 apple, pear, or orange
             Water

DINNER	Ronnie's Broiled Chicken Breasts* Steamed Artichoke* with lemon juice Grated Carrot Salad*, *or* Watercress and Mushroom Salad*
BREAKFAST	½ cup Fruity Oatmeal* (unsweetened) ½ cup skimmed milk Herb tea, unsweetened
LUNCH	Vegetable Pita Pocket* 1 apple, pear, or orange Water
DINNER	Stir-Fried Tofu and Vegetables* ⅓ cup cooked bulgur Frozen Apple Yogurt* Water

Snacks: Crudités* only, 1 cup per day.

Any sudden switch in the caloric intake is a stress to the body, so you should also pay attention to the vitamins and minerals that will help your body handle this new stress. I suggest that, while you're on this diet, you take:

Calcium, 1000 mg daily.

Magnesium, 750 to 1000 mg daily. These are usually taken at bedtime, as they have a calming effect and will promote natural, nondrugged rest.

The B complex: a capsule with 50 mg of each of the B's and 50 mcg of B_{12} and 0.4 mg of folic acid. Inositol, choline, and PABA are usually included. The B vitamins tend to make the body more efficient and seem to sustain the blood sugar, so the dieter does not get quite so frantic or restless.

Vitamin C makes everything work better. Probably at least 1000 to 5000 mg every day, depending upon the state of the bowel movements; if they are soft, cut back.

An all-purpose vitamin capsule with the Recommended Daily Allowance of all the vitamins and minerals, because you have no assurance that the good foods that you are eating have come from well-endowed, nondepleted soil that had everything in it. Chromium, 200 mcg; zinc, 30 mg; and manganese, 15 mg, seem to help the dieter diet.

Suitable aerobic exercise, because it stimulates the production of endorphins, will reduce hunger.

Diet 2: Teens-on-the-Run Diet

These dishes can be made quickly; they taste good and can be carried with you. Think of your ancient relatives running after animals in the wild or over the plains. They ate mainly raw vegetables, fruit in season, and lean meats—they had no dairy products because of the difficulty in milking a deer on the run—some nuts and seeds, and that was about it. Try to imitate them as closely as possible. Nibble, nibble. Run, run. See if eating an apple or a whole-grain sandwich just before some boring class helps to keep you awake.

These foods all provide the protein, fiber, and complex carbohydrates that we all need. Just to be sure, take a multipurpose vitamin and mineral capsule as a supplement. Calcium and magnesium at bedtime is a good idea, too.

BREAKFAST	1 cup plain low-fat yogurt, or 1–2 hard-boiled eggs 1–2 Bran Muffins* or slices whole-grain toast 1 apple or banana
LUNCH	Peanut Butter and Honey Sandwich* Crudités* 1 apple, pear, or orange Water
DINNER	(to eat at home) Ronnie's Broiled Chicken Breasts* Couscous Steamed broccoli 1 piece fruit of your choice Water
DINNER	(to eat on the run) Tofu Salad Sandwich* or Tofu Quiche* Crudités*

1 apple, pear, or orange
Granola Bar*
Water

BREAKFAST Banana Yogurt Smoothie*
1–2 muffins of your choice* or Granola Bars*

LUNCH Cucumber Cottage Cheese Sandwich*
Crudités*
1 apple, pear, or orange
2 Oatmeal Cookies*
Water

DINNER (to eat at home)
Broiled Salmon Steaks*
Baked Tomatoes*
Steamed new potatoes
Apples with Lime Juice*
Water

DINNER (to eat on the run)
Tuna Salad Pita Pocket*
Crudités*
1 apple, pear, or orange
Granola Bar* or Oatmeal Cookie*
Water

BREAKFAST 1 slice Breakfast Cheesecake*
1 muffin of your choice, or 1–2 slices whole-grain
   toast
1 orange or apple

LUNCH Spinach and Tofu Pita Sandwich*
Crudités*
2 Oatmeal Cookies*
1 orange or peach
Water

DINNER (to eat at home)
Cabbage Soup à la Chinoise*
Whole wheat bread
Tossed green salad with Low-Fat Vinaigrette*
Fruit of your choice
Water

DINNER   (to eat on the run)
                Chinese Chicken Salad* sandwich
                Crudités*
                1 apple, pear, or orange
                Water

Snacks: Your choice from Chapter 4, two a day.

Diet 3: Improved-Complexion Diet

This diet emphasizes vegetables high in vitamin A and the B complex vitamins, and is very low in fat. It also works well for people with allergies. Eating sugary food and nutritionally impoverished bread and cereals does not lead directly to oily skin and acne, but the digestion of these foods is such a stress to the body's enzyme systems, that depletion sets in. The adolescent who is already stressed by his overwhelming hormones has enough to cope with without starving himself on empty foods. Ideally, these nonsense foods should not be available: The soda cracker, for instance, has nothing in it that is good for us; it's all salt, white flour, fat and sugar. Greasy doughnuts and French fries will give most of us pimples, either on our faces or buttocks.

See Chapter 2 for a description of the vitamin and mineral supplements for acne control, but, in general, vitamin A needs to be taken in sufficient amounts to encourage a dryness to the skin. Vitamin A can be toxic to some people, but a heavy dose of 75,000 to 100,000 units a day for a month should not cause side effects and would show you that you are on the right track. If your mouth feels dry, however, you should cut way back on the supplement dosage, but keep concentrating on foods rich in Vitamin A. After the first month you should cut back to a more reasonable maintenance dose, to 10,000 to 20,000 units a day. Zinc helps the A and so does vitamin E. Zinc, 30 to 60 mg a day, and 400 to 800 units of the E every day along with the diet is standard.

BREAKFAST   ¼ cantaloupe
              ½ cup Fruity Oatmeal* (without milk)
              Herb tea, unsweetened

LUNCH	Broccoli Salad* with tofu added, *or* 1 cup Blender Gazpacho* (with no seeds or yogurt garnish) Crudités* 1 pear 2 glasses water
DINNER	Fish Teriyaki*, *or* broiled lean fish filet of your choice ⅓ cup brown rice Spinach and Tangerine Salad* 1 piece fresh fruit 2 glasses water
BREAKFAST	Pineapple Banana Mint Smoothie* Herb tea, unsweetened
LUNCH	Grated Carrot Salad* Crudités* ½ can water-packed tunafish 1 apple 2 glasses water
DINNER	Chicken Noodle *or* Tofu Noodle Soup* Tossed green salad with lemon juice Steamed Artichoke* with lemon juice Oranges with Mint* 2 glasses water
BREAKFAST	Fruit and Sprout Smoothie* Herb tea, unsweetened
LUNCH	Middle Eastern Salad* Crudités* Carrot Apple Drink*
DINNER	Tofu Sprouts Salad* (without sunflower or sesame seeds) Steamed Greens with Vinegar or Lemon Juice* (cook in water instead of oil) Baked Pears* 2 glasses water

Snacks: Crudités*, emphasizing cucumbers, carrots, and greens. Also drink lots of vegetable juices.

Diet 4: Nondairy, Nonwheat Diet for Allergic Teens

This is designed for people with milk and wheat sensitivities. When I started my pediatric practice in the early 1950s it was estimated that one person in 10 was sensitive to dairy products. Now it is believed that one person in two has some trouble with cow's milk. Some of that may be due to the mother's drinking a quart of homogenized/pasteurized milk every day during the pregnancy, and some of it may be that many mothers elected not to nurse their babies. Some of the blame, however, must be laid on the pediatrician who felt it was important to start solid foods in the first few weeks of life! We now know this is not a good practice and probably is such a stress to the baby that he became sensitized to all those foods introduced too early. It makes the babies allergy-prone.

If you have ever had a couple of ear infections or a strep throat you are probably allergic to dairy products. If you have gas and some sloppy bowel movements, you are probably sensitive to wheat. Especially if you like it.

I see bedwetting, nosebleeds, susceptibility to infections, pimples, gas, and arthritis as a sign of sensitivity to any food. If you have any symptom from fatigue and insomnia to rashes and migraines, try this diet for about three weeks and see if you feel better. You might get bored with it, but try hard to persevere, especially if you feel good. You'll find it is worth it. Remember, when you drink milk you are depriving a calf.

If you find this type of allergen-free diet is good for you, you may find that you can have some wheat or milk on a rotational basis, but only once every four to five days, without falling apart. For example, if I don't drink coffee, I can eat a cookie every once in a while without getting a headache. If I eat cheese occasionally, I am okay, but if I drink a glass of milk too, I will have a nosebleed in twenty minutes.

You live in your body, so *you* have to figure it out. Remember, the skin tests used by allergists are practically worthless for testing for food sensitivities; don't waste your money.

Some have found that the whey protein in milk does not cause any special symptoms, since the allergen-villain is casein.

You could try the whey milks on the market, although be careful of those sweetened with corn sweeteners, which can cause trouble.

Health food stores are now catering to the demand for wheat- and dairy-free foods. There are rice cakes and other foods less likely to cause trouble. Rye bread usually has some wheat in it, although Russian rye might be okay. I have found that the Spicer Company's snack foods are safe and do not seem to arouse the allergy potential despite the fact that they contain wheat and whey. They treat the basic grains they use in such a way that they are broken down in the intestines to a nonallergic form. (For more information, call Spicer's International: 1/800/824-3196.)

Because dairy products supply much of our calcium needs, it would be wise to take 1000 mg of calcium daily. Zinc, 30 mg, seems to help the intestines digest foods down to their nonallergic parts. Many people find that they need to take digestive enzymes to help this process. Those with yeast infection often have food allergies and low thyroid function. (See *Dr. Lendon Smith's Low-Stress Diet*, New York: McGraw-Hill, 1985.)

BREAKFAST	¾ cup Fruity Oatmeal*, without milk (you may substitute soy or goat's milk) 6 ounces orange juice Herb tea
LUNCH	1 cup Gazpacho* (no yogurt for garnish) Crudités* 2 nonwheat crackers 1 apple, orange, or pear Water
DINNER	Poached Filet of Sole with Tomato Puree* ½ cup brown rice Steamed broccoli Sliced melon
BREAKFAST	1–2 soft-boiled eggs 2 rye or other nonwheat crackers ½ grapefruit (*or* ¼ cantaloupe) Herb tea

LUNCH   1 cup Lentil Salad* (do not use yogurt in the dress-
               ing; substitute half cooking liquid from the lentils,
               half lemon juice)
               Crudités*
               2 nonwheat crackers
               1 apple, orange, or pear
               Water

DINNER   1 cup Black Beans*
               2–3 corn tortillas
               Spinach Salad* (no yogurt in dressing; substitute
               lemon juice)
               Oranges with Mint*
               Water

BREAKFAST   ¾ cup Hot Mixed Grains Cereal* (without wheat
               flakes), no milk (can substitute soy milk or goat's
               milk), or ¾ cup cold nonwheat cereal (see ap-
               proved list, page 154), moistened with apple
               juice, soy milk, or goat's milk
               6 ounces fruit juice
               Herb tea

LUNCH   1 cup Chinese Chicken Salad* (omit yogurt in
               dressing; substitute ¼ cup lemon juice)
               Crudités*
               2 nonwheat crackers
               1 apple, pear, or orange
               Water

DINNER   Stir-Fried Tofu and Vegetables*
               ½ cup cooked millet
               Oriental Sprouts Salad* (use vegetable stock, no
               yogurt, in dressing)
               Poached Bananas* (omit yogurt)
               Water

Snacks: Emphasize Crudités*, fruit and vegetable juices,
frozen ice pops (not those containing yogurt). Caution: Baked
goods and candies often contain milk or milk products and
wheat products.

Diet 5: Weight-Gain Diet for Boys (and Girls, Too)

This diet emphasizes calories and complex carbohydrates. Until just recently it was thought that to make muscles one had to *eat* muscles; in other words, a high-protein, high-meat diet was recommended. This almost makes sense, but the emphasis on meat is not the best way. If about 20 percent of the diet is high-quality protein, the muscle and tissues and blood will get their share. Vegetarians' diets make perfectly good muscles for them. The glycogen stored in the muscles gives endurance and energy; exercise and male hormone contribute to the size and bulk. We all have seen Schwartzenegger's muscles. He is male, he has a balanced diet but he *keeps* the muscles there with exercise, and smiting and smoting.

I started a body building club when I was about 13. A friend and I lifted weights until we got tired and sweaty. It did build up our torsos and biceps; so we did look better, but we had forgotten to run or bike to train the muscles for endurance, so we weren't really stronger than before. Weight lifting and static exercise build muscle size and bulk; muscles from running are usually long and thin; swimming muscles seem to be more supple. Just a few years ago, coaches told their athletes just to run if they were runners and only swim if they were aiming for water sports medals. Now we know that any and all exercise that uses a muscle will tend to enlarge the muscle and a variety of exercises will help all-around strength and endurance. It looks like a variety of exercises, walking, running, swimming, weight lifting, are all good to build up the muscles and hence the good-looking body. Start slow and build up.

Some athletes find that carbohydrate loading before a long run is helpful since more glycogen gets stored in the muscles and hence more usable stored fuel is available at the time of need. (Many runners in the New York Marathon gather for a spaghetti dinner the night before the race.) This does not work, though, for everyone. You should try a number of different food combinations before deciding what's best for you. But stay away from too much meat!

Supplements that would help your body on this diet are mainly the B complex vitamins, maybe about 50 mg of each of the B's, and 50 mcg of B_{12} and 0.4 mg of folic acid. Vitamin C helps everything. If you are eating a lot and stay thin and washed-out looking, you should have a thorough medical checkup. If all is in order, you might ask the doctor to give you a few B complex shots or at least B_{12} injections (twice a week for 3 weeks) and see if that improves your digestion and absorption.

BREAKFAST	Double serving Fruity Oatmeal* Banana Yogurt Smoothie*
LUNCH	2 Black Bean Burritos* ½ avocado, sliced, with Tofu Mayonnaise* 2–4 Oatmeal Cookies* 1 piece fruit 1 cup skim milk
DINNER	Spinach Lasagne* (1–2 helpings) Tossed green salad with Yogurt Vinaigrette* 1–2 slices whole-grain bread Peach Cobbler* 1 cup skim milk
BREAKFAST	Mushroom Omelette* 2 Bran Muffins* ½ cantaloupe
LUNCH	2 "Chili Dogs"* 1–2 pieces Cornbread* Carrot Apple Salad* 2 Granola Bars* 1 piece fruit 1 cup skim milk
DINNER	Corn Chowder* (1–2 servings) Potato Bean Tacos* (3–4) ½ avocado, sliced Spinach Salad* Carob Ice Pops (recipe on page 92) 1 cup skim milk

BREAKFAST	1 cup granola* with 1 sliced banana 1 cup milk 1–2 Bran Muffins* 8 ounces orange juice
LUNCH	Minestrone* (1–2 helpings) Curried Brown Rice Salad* 2 slices whole-grain bread 2 ounces cheese 1 slice Breakfast Cheesecake* 1 cup skim milk
DINNER	Minestrone* (1–2 helpings) Spaghetti with Tofu Tomato Sauce*, *or* Homemade Pizza* 1–2 slices whole-grain bread Broccoli Salad* Banana Yogurt Ice Cream* 2 Oatmeal Cookies* 1 cup skim milk

Snacks: Three to four a day, your choice, from Chapter 4.

CHAPTER 8

Exercise Is the Only Diet That Works

What I'm about to tell you might sound like bad news to some of you and good news to others: *Diets without exercise don't work.*

When you diet you put yourself into a state of semistarvation; that's why you're always in a bad mood. You think it's because you can't have ice cream, but really it's because your body is being deprived of food; you are keeping yourself in a state of constant, intense hunger and setting yourself up for a binge. The hunger accumulates, but you can't afford to listen to your body telling you it needs to eat, because you are on a diet. So eventually you become deaf to your body's messages, and, if the dieting goes on long enough, even when you go off of it you never know when you are really hungry and when you're not. All the normal internal signals have become useless as guides to when and how much you should eat. That's why bingeing usually goes along with dieting.

It's natural that the body should want to compensate for its caloric deprivation. It is as if famine had set in. Our physiology has not evolved too much over the years, and our ancestors, who lived with the constant threat of famine, were often forced to consume as many calories at one time as they could. But our ancestors were a lot more active than we are, and their calories were never the empty kind that we are used to consuming. No Cokes in the olden days.

Here's another reason why dieting doesn't work, and in fact becomes self-defeating in the long run. Dieting, by depriving the body of calories over a long period, eventually begins to act as a signal that tells the body to *turn down its metabolic rate* so that it can store more energy. This slows the rate of weight loss, and when you resume your normal eating habits, because your metabolism is now slower you will actually gain back more than you lost!!! So dieting, in effect, leads to a tendency to *gain*.

If you are taking appetite suppressants like amphetamines, the results are just the same, and sometimes worse. You might think that the diet pills are suppressing your appetite, but what they are actually doing is increasing your metabolic rate—which makes you feel speedy. When you go off the amphetamines, your metabolic rate drops back and your tendency to gain is even greater. That's so upsetting that you go back onto the diet pills. Eventual result: addiction.

Feeling totally discouraged by all this? Well, there is an answer, and it can be a lot more fun than dieting: *exercise*.

Science has now proven that activity is much more important than food in regulating fatness. Animals always grow fatter when they are not allowed to exercise: you normally put on a few pounds in winter, when you are more sedentary. (Also, you tend to eat more when you are sedentary.) For human beings, the inactive life we have grown to lead is very recent, and it is as abnormal as caging an animal.

The reason exercise is a more effective method of weight control than dieting is because sustained physical activity eventually increases your amount of muscle tissue, which alters your body chemistry and speeds up your metabolism so that you burn calories more efficiently *even while you sleep!*

Here's how it works. Thinness and fatness actually have more to do with the percentage of fat you have than with your actual weight. We all need to have a certain amount of fat, and storage of fat is a natural bodily function. Fat people are just overly proficient at it; they burn calories less easily. But the reason for this is that fat does not require energy. Muscles, on the other hand, do. *Muscles burn calories*. They are full of special enzymes whose purpose is burning up calories quickly, and they need lots of calories because movement is our most energy-demanding bodily function. Muscles burn 90 percent of the calories burned in the body. So the greater your muscle mass, the more calories you will burn all the time. That is, if the muscles are in tone.

That's another reason why dieting is self-defeating. When you diet you usually reduce your muscle mass, another reason why you lower your metabolism. Even if you lose pounds, you lose muscle along with the fat, and that does nothing to improve your shape.

Aerobic exercise increases the number of the calorie-burning enzymes located in your muscle cells. It increases the burning of fats and calories throughout the day, and not just when we are deliberately exercising. In fact, relatively few calories are burned during the physical activity itself (so choose the exercise you *like*, not just the one the charts say requires the most energy). It is the cumulative effect that works to transform your body into an independent, self-regulating organism. Exercise yourself down to a low fat level and a high muscle-tone level, and you will never have to count calories again, as long as you stay active.

Think Enzymes and Muscle Tone, Not Weight

When you begin a regular exercise program you might be surprised and dismayed to find that you are not losing weight. That is, the scales don't look encouraging. In fact, you may gain a few pounds. Because *muscle is heavier than fat*. But soon you will see that your shape is beginning to change; and that's what you wanted in the first place. What you have gained is lean body mass. By exercising, you are reducing the fat stores that are inside the muscle, and making your muscles long, lean, and firm. If you rely on dieting only, you will not lose anything but the fat under your skin, and the shape of your body will remain the same.

Spot reducing doesn't work either, because the caloric demand is small when only one set of muscles is exercised. Spot reducing just results in a larger muscle with the same fat deposits on top. When large sets of muscles are exercised, fat is drawn from all over the body to meet the muscles' energy requirements. The more muscle you have, the more energy you need to burn, and the more enzymes you have to burn it.

Aerobic Exercise

The kind of exercise that results in this overall change in muscle tone and metabolism is called *aerobic* exercise. It is steady exercise—uninterrupted for at least 12 minutes—which makes the muscles work hard enough to require lots of oxygen. The goal is to increase your heartbeat to what is called a "training heart rate" by exercising your muscles steadily for at least 12 to 20 minutes (preferably longer), depending on the sport. When you do this kind of exercise regularly—three days a week or more—you increase your muscle mass so that your body burns more calories at all times.

How to Determine Your Training Heart Rate. First determine your "resting heart rate." Using a sweep second hand, take your pulse for six seconds; multiply this by 10. If you were between counts on the sixth second, say six and seven, your resting heart rate will be 65. Use Dr. Kenneth Cooper's* formula: Subtract your age in years from 220 (this value, 220, is supposed to be the maximum heart rate for an optimally trained athlete). 65% of this would be your minimum training rate and 85% of this would be your maximum training heart rate. Thus at age 15, your maximum heart rate would be 205, your minimum rate during exercise to produce benefits would be (205 × .65) or 133 beats/minute and your maximum personal training rate would be (205 × 0.85) or 174 beats/minute and it would be best not to exceed this. During exercise, take your pulse. It should be between 133 and 174 beats per minute.

You should choose an exercise that uses all of the muscles fully, and that is not a stop-and-go sport; 15 minutes of jogging

* Cooper, Kenneth H., M.D., and Mildred. *Aerobics for Women*, Bantam, New York, 1982.

is more effective for maintaining muscle tone and body weight than two hours of tennis (unless you are Martina Navratilova). The activity must be continuous; you can't break it up and exercise twice during the day for 6 minutes. And of course, more than 12 minutes will increase your muscle tone and metabolism even more. Devoting more time does more for you than exercising harder. But exercising six days a week for a short time, say 12 minutes, does more for you than exercising three days a week for 30 minutes. Certain aerobic exercises require more time to work up to the heart rate necessary for long-term metabolic changes. The benefits will be lost altogether if you exercise *less* than three days a week. For *losing* weight you should increase exercise time to 30 minutes.

Choosing an Aerobic Exercise

The most important thing to consider when choosing your form of exercise is: What do you like? If running makes your legs hurt too much, don't run. If you hate getting your hair wet, swimming isn't for you. If you like sociable sports and fresh air don't do calisthenics alone in your basement. Sometimes you won't love a sport at first but will grow to love it, because it will make you feel so good. You must be able to assimilate your activity into your lifestyle. If you are short on time, then the shortest forms of exercise with the greatest efficiency are the ones to consider. If you are more likely to be conscientious if you choose something that isn't solitary, look into aerobic dance classes. They are offered everywhere, and there is something comforting about all those people struggling through the exercises with you. Any exercise may seem like torture at first, if you aren't in shape, but after a while they become addictive, and this is the kind of addiction to seek.

Indeed, exercising produces a psychological high greater than any drug, and will fill up that boredom space you might otherwise deal with by bingeing and watching television. The more you exercise the less likely you are to overeat, because you become so aware of your body and its signals. That's why exercise is the best diet there is.

No matter what you choose, always begin by doing the minimum, and gradually work up to more. Stretch out for three to five minutes before and afterward, to warm up and cool down. Don't push yourself too hard or you may eventually give up. If you are overweight or underweight, or generally feel that you are a clod, as I did during my teenage years, it may be difficult for you to begin a sport because you don't want the other kids to see you in a bathing suit, or in gym shorts, or trying to struggle around the track. If it is just too mortifying for you, choose something that you can do in private, like cycling (either outside or on a stationary bicycle) or jumping rope.

Everything takes time. If you are out of shape, the first time you swim you'll feel like you're going to drown. So swim the minimum; then, every couple of days, add another lap or two. Soon you'll be swimming a mile. If you have a lot of body fat, even though you feel self-conscious in a bathing suit, swimming may be the easiest sport for you, because fat floats, and you won't strain any muscles or jar your body, as you would, say, jogging. Remember, once you are in the water nobody sees you. Also, when you begin to look around the locker room you will notice how many different kinds of bodies there are, and you may begin to like your own. But if you just don't like getting wet, riding a stationary regular bicycle might be perfect for you.

When you begin to do strenuous exercise, the first 10 minutes are the most excruciating: you get out of breath, you ache if you're doing aerobics or a jarring sport. But after those ten minutes you get a second wind and your heart beats comfortably at an elevated rate. Then you can go on for another 10 to 20 minutes or longer and get the maximum out of your exercise. So stick it out. After a month your body will be dependent on this kind of activity, and you will feel added benefits like better sleep, sounder digestion, and a good nature.

An Aerobic Exercise for You

There should be something here for you. Rather than decide on one right away, try a few of these and see which one you like the best. If you like a few of them, by all means vary your activity. You will be exercising different muscles and the overall effect will be even better. I have noted the minimum times required to reach your training heart rate, but remember, more is better.

Begin, though, with short-range goals which you can increase every day. If you are jumping rope, for example, work up to 100 jumps without stopping during the first two weeks to a month. Then work up to 15 minutes without stopping during the next two months, and finally set your goal at 30 minutes.

And, once you've picked your activity, turn to Chapter 10's "Low-Calorie Diet for Noncompetitors" to get the proper nutritional support for your new lifestyle.

Walking. America's most popular athletic pursuit. Minimum time 20 minutes, and you should increase to 40 minutes for the best results. Walk long and briskly, swing your arms, pull in your stomach, take long strides. The effect of your endurance will be as great as that of cycling or swimming.

Running (or Jogging). Minimum 15 minutes. Beginners should walk before you run. That is, start and stop, walking briskly between each run. As your wind improves, increase the proportion of running to walking, until you are running the entire time.

This is one of the hardest for non-exercisers, because your legs will get quite sore at the beginning. Run only three times a week until your muscles stop aching, and never two days in a row. It is also quite a difficult one for very overweight people, because of the jarring effect and the strain on joints. So it might not be the one for you. It also may be intimidating for women with large breasts, because of this same jarring. But don't despair; you can buy a special athletic bra, which has much more support.

This sport trains faster than any other, with the exception of cross-country skiing and rowing, and is very good for quick weight loss. Remember, you don't have to be a racer. You can run anywhere, around the neighborhood, around a lake, around a track, even around your basement. And you can run slowly or fast. It is a nice social sport (once you reach your second wind), as well as a fulfilling solitary activity.

Bicycling (Outdoor or Stationary).   Minimum time 20 minutes. Nutritionists and doctors are turning more and more to the bicycle as a means of exercising their patients. You really work when you pedal. If you use a stationary bicycle, put on a pair of headphones and listen to music as you go. Outside, you should wear a helmet; no room for the earphones. Bicycling is easier on the legs and joints than running and jumping sports, and is more comfortable for big-busted women. I recommend it highly for the overweight person and the klutz. Most of us know how to ride a bicycle, and that's all the skill you need for this sport. You can ride around the block, along city streets, country roads, on bicycle paths along rivers or around lakes. You can ride with friends or alone. Cycling is a good activity for the entire family; everyone can go at his or her own pace, but you are always somehow together. When you begin, try to ride a mile at a time, and work up to 5 miles over eight weeks time. Then go as far as you have time for.

Swimming.   Minimum time 20 minutes. Swimming, like biking, is a lifelong sport. It is easy on your joints and bones and exercises all the skeletal muscles in your body. It is almost impossible to injure yourself while swimming. It is adaptable; you can swim laps in a pool, distances in lakes or the ocean. Synchronized swimming is one of the most strenuous of sports, while at the same time being more social than lap swimming. This sport is a good one for teens too stocky, small, or short for competitive sports like basketball and football. Once you're in the water, your size is irrelevant.

It's easy to learn to swim, once you overcome your fear of the water. A qualified instructor can teach you in just a few lessons. When you begin swimming, swim as far as you can the first day, then add a lap or a few more minutes every time. You can vary your strokes between crawl, breast stroke, and backstroke (side-stroke isn't strenuous enough). Sing to yourself as you swim so you don't get bored.

Jumping Rope.   Minimum time 12 to 15 minutes. This exercise can be addictive and is one of the most exertive. You may not have done it since elementary school playground days, but when you take it up again it may bring back fond memories. These associations, however, should not discourage boys from jumping rope. Men have used jumping rope as a training exercise for other sports (boxing, football, etc.) for years.

You can jump rope in any space larger than a closet, which makes this a good travel sport. Listen to music as you skip, or talk with friends. If you feel klutzy at first, go through the skipping motion for a while without the rope; then gradually begin using the rope. It is actually not jumping, but skipping, one foot after another, that you want to be doing, as you can keep this up for a longer time and it isn't as jarring. This is an exercise that overweight and big-busted people might want to steer clear of.

Dance. Minimum time 15 minutes. All dance is terrific aerobic exercise as long as you dance continuously and vigorously (a slow fox trot would not do the trick). Ballet, modern, folk, and tap will all give you a good workout. And of course, aerobic dance, which has become such a rage in recent years, is terrific. You must choose your class carefully, though, especially if you are a beginner, because some teachers work their classes so rigorously, not really considering the various levels of the students, that you might become discouraged. If you are very overweight, look around for classes geared for overweight people.

Dance classes are a good choice for people who don't like exercising alone. The fact that you have signed up for a course and somebody is paying for it can be very motivating.

Cross-Country Skiing. Minimum time 15 minutes. This is one of the most demanding sports. Like swimming, it uses a great number of muscles. But it's more exhausting—and exhilarating. The problem, of course, is that it's not something you can do every day, unless you live in the country, and then you can only do it in winter. It's best to do this one in conjunction with something else.

Jumping Jacks. Minimum time 12 to 15 minutes. Jumping jacks, like jumping rope, is one of the calisthenic exercises that can work your heart up to a training rate in a very short time. It's one of the exercises to do with music, perhaps with friends, as part of a longer workout. It is difficult for overweight and big-busted people.

Rowing. Minimum time 15 minutes. This is one of the most strenuous of aerobic sports. You can row by yourself or with a friend, or on a rowing team. If you like being on a lake or a river, this is a sport to consider. It will build your muscle tone, especially arms, stomach, and back. Boys who feel scrawny might benefit from this one.

Figure Skating. Minimum time 20 minutes. This can be a highly demanding aerobic exercise, if you skate steadily. Try to find rinks or ponds that aren't too crowded, so that you can give yourself a workout without running into people. When you concentrate on your form you use your stomach and buttock muscles as well as your leg muscles, and the overall toning effect is quite good.

Roller Skating. Minimum time 20 minutes. As with figure skating, when you skate quickly, but steadily, with control, over a long period of time, you get aerobic benefits. This is another good one to do with friends, and you will probably find that 20 minutes isn't enough.

Canoeing and Kayaking. Minimum time 15 minutes. Like rowing, these can be highly aerobic if you are not just paddling along, but really working over 15 minutes (you will no doubt want to be out there a lot longer). Of course you have to be near water if you're going to choose this as your activity.

Mini-Trampoline. Minimum time 15 minutes. Trampoline work has much the same benefits as jumping jacks and jumping rope, with the added advantage of not being jarring. You must use your entire body, swinging your arms, bending your legs as you hit the trampoline, pushing yourself up vigorously. Another one that's fun to do to music.

Aerobic and Anaerobic Exercises and Sports

These activities are aerobic *if* they involve continuous exertion for at least 20 minutes. For the most part they are not considered aerobic, but can be excellent for muscle toning and stretching; for the best aerobic benefits, supplement them with something from the above group.

Stop-and-Go Exercises

Alpine Skiing.   This can be aerobic if you ski hard enough to raise your heart rate and keep it up for 15 minutes or more. You need long runs for this.

Basketball.   If you keep moving on the court this can be one of the best aerobic exercises.

Handball, Squash, and Racquetball.   These sports can be highly aerobic if you are well matched with your opponents and have long, strenuous rallies. Handball is less likely to be aerobic than squash and racquetball.

Tennis.   This can be aerobic if the rallies are long and you hit the ball hard and far, so that you and your opponent run a lot.

Badminton and Volleyball.   These can be aerobic if they are power sports, not the kind of Sunday sports that you play on the beach. Usually, though, there is too much starting and stopping for them to be considered aerobic.

Field Hockey, Lacrosse, and Soccer.   These field sports can be aerobic for players in forward positions if activity is constant for over 20 minutes. For fullback positions, and definitely for the goalie, these are stop-start sports.

Calisthenics.   Calisthenics are muscle-toning exercises like sit-ups, push-ups, leg lifts, and deep knee bends. They are very good for firming the body and making you more flexible, but they are not really aerobic exercises. Jumping jacks and running in place are aerobic calisthenics and are often combined with other calisthenic exercises in workouts, for a marvelous overall effect on the body.

Karate, Judo, Aikido, Kung Fu, Tae Kwon Do. These Far Eastern martial arts can be aerobic if your training sessions are intense workouts, two hours long. Beginners would not get aerobic benefits for some time. Matches are stop-and-go.

Fencing. This can be aerobic during training, but is a stop-and-go exercise during matches.

Water-Skiing. This can be aerobic if you ski steadily and move in and out of the wake a lot.

Nonaerobic Short-Duration Exercise

Football
Weightlifting
Sprinting
Isometrics
Gymnastics
Track-and-field sports (except running)

Advice to the Nonathlete

This is the category I fell into when I was your age. Gym class was agony to me. I only wish I had had the kind of information you have now, to get me going then on an exercise program.

Boys. Your biggest embarrassment is probably that you are (1) too skinny and uncoordinated, (2) too fat and uncoordinated, or (3) just plain uncoordinated.

Choose an exercise, then, that doesn't rely so much on coordination. Jogging or fast walking, riding a bicycle, swimming, and calisthenics are all suitable for the klutz. These are sports that can be enjoyed alone as well as with friends. I would say that one of the best all-around aerobic exercises, one that will spare you the embarrassment of feeling you look too thin or fat, or seem too uncoordinated, is bicycling. You don't have to be a racer, and you don't have to find the steepest hills in town; just pedal steadily for a half hour every day, around the lake or along a country lane.

Girls. Your sources of embarrassment don't differ too much from the boys', although more of you are afraid to be seen in gym clothes or a bathing suit because you think you're too fat than because you think you're scrawny.

Choose exercises that aren't too jarring if you are over-weight. An exercise class that stresses stretching and building muscle tone, with enough time devoted to aerobics to get your heartbeat up, but not so much that you don't want to come back the next day, is the kind of class to look for. Swimming might be more suitable than jogging, as it's easier on the body. If you can transcend the embarrassment you might feel about being seen in a bathing suit (wear a robe to the pool's edge, then throw it off and jump in), you might find yourself becoming quickly addicted to this activity. Riding a stationary bicycle and cycling are two marvelous forms of exercise that will build up endurance and muscle tone without bringing attention to your body or emphasizing any kind of competition. You can bike with friends and talk as you pedal.

CHAPTER 9

Eating to Win

Feeding Your Muscles: The Myth of the High-Protein Diet

Before I knew about nutrition I used to recommend the same steak-and-eggs training breakfast that coaches recommended for their athletes. Now I know better, and so do the professional athletes and sports nutrition doctors. There is nothing worse for peak performance, whether you are a football star or a 15-minutes-a-day jogger, than the steak-and-eggs training meal. Athletes do not need to eat high-protein diets. In fact, they need to cut down on protein and emphasize complex carbohydrates. Athletes like Martina Navratilova, Jimmy Connors, Stan Smith, and Fred Stolle will convince you, if I can't, that complex carbohydrates increase energy, endurance, and sports performance.

Remember, we are thinking *muscles*. Muscles are fueled by carbohydrates, which are stored in the muscles as a substance called *glycogen*. When muscles work they burn the glycogen; it must be resupplied several times during the day. That's just what a high-carbohydrate diet will do; it will double the amount of glycogen in your muscles and increase your energy supply.

These must be *complex* carbohydrates, like grains, cereals, potatoes, and pasta. I'm not talking about candy bars and soft drinks. Complex carbohydrates are the key to regulating your metabolism and burning fats. Simple carbohydrates—sugar—stimulate the pancreas to produce high levels of insulin, which tells the body to make and store fat, and makes you get hungry more often. Sugar increases the level of fats (triglycerides) in the blood, which reduces your athletic endurance and puts you, even at your young age, at high risk for cardiovascular disease.

Protein serves as a highly inefficient energy supply, and an unbalanced high-protein diet can reverse the effects of exercise and can actually be harmful for the athlete. Contrary to much popular opinion, high-protein diets build fatter bodies, not bigger muscles, and they lead to quick fatigue and poor performance. The steak-and-eggs diet is not only a high-protein diet, it is a high-*fat* diet, much higher in calories than a high-carbohydrate diet. That's why we're finding more and more vegetarians among the Olympic gold medalists and other professional athletes. At any rate, it isn't necessary to eat red meat to get high-quality protein. You find the same amino acids in poultry, fish, low-fat dairy products, eggs, and balanced combinations of grains and legumes.

In addition to protein's inefficiency in providing energy for the athlete, there are other reasons why a high-protein diet can be downright dangerous. When you eat excess protein, your body is tremendously taxed: your liver is forced to work much harder in order to digest the large amount of protein, and your kidneys are strained by the extra water required to wash out the excess. To make matters even worse, because the body produces so much urine in the process, you also excrete many vital minerals necessary for, among other things, peak athletic performance. The potassium you lose helps control muscle temperature, blood flow, and nerve conduction; the calcium you lose is vital for strong bones and proper muscle function; and the magnesium helps regulate muscle contraction and the conversion of carbohydrates into energy.

A high-protein diet which is low in carbohydrates can be devastating, over time, to muscle tissue. The brain, as well as your muscles, is fueled by carbohydrates, which also produce a sugar called glucose: brain food. If there aren't enough carbohydrates in your diet, the body will use protein for glucose production, when the protein should be spending its time repairing muscle tissue and replacing other cells. So your muscles can eventually degenerate and lose their tone. Result: reduction in lean body mass, just the thing you were trying to increase by running all those miles.

The other risk is dehydration, as your body uses up a lot of water digesting all that protein and getting rid of the toxins. Which brings me to the subject of the most important drink for athletes:

H_2O

Inadequate hydration is the major cause of poor performance in sports. Sports nutritionists say that water is the athlete's single most important nutrient. The body needs water to regulate its temperature through perspiration, to rid itself of toxic wastes through urination, and to maintain proper blood pressure. Water supplies the muscles and organs with oxygen and nutrients, and water is vital for the energy-supplying chemical reactions that occur in the muscles.

Thirst is not an adequate indication of how much water an active person needs. You need to force it. That's not too difficult if you begin to replace soft drinks and "sports drinks" with water. When Jimmy Connors began to do that, and to change his pregame steak-and-potatoes meal to spaghetti, he won at Wimbledon.

Athletes should drink at least one pint of water before exercise or competition, and should continually drink during competition. *Eat to Win* nutrition doctor Robert Haas recommends three or more glasses three hours prior to sports events, two glasses 60 to 15 minutes before, and at least two glasses per hour while performing. After your event you should weigh yourself and drink two cups of water for every pound you've lost. You may have to run to the bathroom more often, but you will perform better. The more active you are, the more water you need.

The idea that athletes should take salt tablets is a myth that couldn't be further from the truth. Salt tablets are dangerous for anybody, and *especially* athletes. They distort the ratio of salt and water in the body and interfere with the body's sweating mechanism. Salt pulls all that water you now know the athlete needs right out of the muscles, and too much can harm the kidneys. If you are worried about losing salt, drink more water.

And water means *water*. A little fresh lemon or fresh orange juice mixed in is okay (2 tablespoons per cup of water), but forget about "sports drinks" like Gatorade. The sugar and salt in these drinks actually pulls water away from the muscles. And that sugar can't get to your muscles anyway, because digestion stops during strenuous physical activity.

What to Eat

Active people (that means all of you), then, should forget what they've been told all their lives about potatoes, grains, pasta, and (whole-grain) bread. These foods are not "fattening," and they should constitute 65 percent of your daily caloric intake. This should be great news to most of you. Spaghetti, the kind you'll find in Chapter 11, and pizza, the kind Martha Rose makes, can go back on your list of "thinning" foods.

Grains are one of the best sources there are for complex carbohydrates. They will also supply you with lots of fiber and vitamins. The roughage is great for your digestive tract, and because grains require a lot of chewing, you will eat more slowly and won't overeat.

Among the nutrients important for athletic performance are potassium, magnesium, and thiamine. Potassium, abundant in bananas, dried fruits, nuts, orange juice, and potatoes, helps regulate the water balance in your body and catalyzes the release of energy and other muscle-cell activities. Insufficient potassium causes muscle fatigue and weakness. Magnesium, abundant in almonds and cashews, meat and fish, milk, whole grains, and dark, leafy greens, is necessary for proper muscle contraction and relaxation, as well as energy release. Thiamine helps your body to burn carbohydrates. Good sources of thiamine include whole-grain breads and cereals, milk, eggs, and organ meats.

Women have greater iron needs than men, especially if they are involved in contact sports, like basketball, martial arts, and jogging (which jars like contact sports). This is because women suffer hidden blood loss from bruising. Some foods rich in iron are dried beans (eat up to 7 cups a week), fresh fruits, grains, broccoli, brussels sprouts, and leafy green vegetables like spinach. Eating vitamin C–enriched foods along with iron-rich foods will help you absorb the iron. Have an orange with your spinach salad.

Calcium and riboflavin (vitamin B_2) are also important nutrients for active women, and I recommend supplements. Riboflavin maximizes the metabolism of protein, fat, and carbohydrates. Calcium needs to be supplemented because the body draws it from the bones when it becomes low (this always happens around the time of your period). If you eat too much protein, so much calcium will be lost that not even supplements will be able to replace it. And don't get hooked into the skinny look or you'll have no stamina at all.

Men who are in training and need to gain weight should increase not their protein intake but their consumption of complex carbohydrates: more potatoes, more whole-grain bread. If you are in intensive training you may have to consume over 6,000 calories a day. But avoid fats. Eat lots of Martha Rose's high-carbohydrate snacks (in Chapter 4).

Wrestlers and participants in other weight-control sports often have severe nutritional problems because of fasting to "make weight." These athletes and their coaches need to review their attitudes about weight control, and their practices. Fasting depletes athletes of carbohydrate stores and water necessary for peak performance. If the athletes also take diuretics and cathartics they deplete their bodies of the minerals necessary for muscle function. They go into their matches thickheaded and lacking in strength and endurance. The notion that wrestlers perform best at their lowest weight is a myth. The crash dieting they routinely subject themselves to can even stunt their growth.

Remember:

- The steak and eggs breakfast will reduce your ability to perform well.
- Complex carbohydrates (grains, pasta, potatoes) increase energy, endurance, and sports performance.
- Consuming sugar causes you to be hungry more often and reduces athletic endurance.
- Protein does not increase your energy supply, and, if eaten in too-great amounts, can reverse the effects of exercise and be harmful to the athlete.
- High-protein diets build fatter bodies, not bigger muscles.
- Eating too much protein can result in dehydration and loss of important minerals such as potassium, calcium, and magnesium.
- "Sports drinks" and salt pills have the opposite effect than that they are reputed to have on athletes: they rob energy and nutrients.
- *Water* is the athlete's single most important nutrient.

10 Nutritional Guidelines for Teenage Athletes and Exercising Nonathletes

1. Reduce the proportion of fats in your diet to 20 to 25 percent of your daily caloric intake.
2. Reduce consumption of protein, especially red meat, to 15 to 20 percent of your daily caloric intake.
3. Reduce intake of sugar.
4. Increase consumption of *complex carbohydrates* (grains, cereals, potatoes, pasta) to 65 percent of your daily caloric intake.
5. Never eat a high-fat, high-protein meal on the day of a competition, or even the day before (the steak-and-eggs training breakfast is out).
6. Drink as much water as possible—at least eight glasses per day. *Replace all soft drinks and sports drinks with water,* preferably bottled spring water.

7. Reduce salt intake to a minimum. Do not take salt tablets; they distort the ratio of salt and water in the body and can cause dehydration and mineral loss.

8. Get lots of the following vitamins and minerals: *potassium, magnesium, thiamine, B complex, B₁₂, folic acid,* and *vitamin C.*

9. Women athletes get lots of the above, plus *calcium, riboflavin,* and *iron.*

10. If you need to gain weight (especially men in training), increase consumption of complex carbohydrates, not protein or fat. And *never* fast or take diuretics or cathartics to make your weight for sports like wrestling.

CHAPTER 10

Maintenance Diets for Athletes

No matter what your sport is, the following menus will provide you with a diet low in fat and high in complex carbohydrates, vitamins, and minerals. This is muscle food, and it happens that muscle food is also good brain food. The diets will not only improve your performance on the playing field, but also in the classroom.

Main Maintenance Diet

These menus are suitable for all active people, whether morning jogger or high school basketball captain. For those of you whose workout needs require more calories, foods whose amounts can be increased are noted.

All asterisked recipes (*) are included, along with general instructions for cooking beans, grains, and pasta, in Chapter 11. See page 194 for explanation of nutrition key.

Day 1

BREAKFAST	1 cup cereal (either from recipes in this book or recommended list on pp. 154–155)	Complex carbohydrate ++ Calcium ++ Potassium + Vitamin C +

½ cup skim milk
1 banana
6 ounces fruit juice

LUNCH	Cucumber Cottage Cheese Spread* on whole wheat bread Crudités* 1 apple 1 cup skim milk	Complex carbohydrate ++ Calcium ++ Fiber + Potassium +
DINNER	Spaghetti with Tomato Sauce and Parmesan* Tossed green salad with Low-Fat Vinaigrette* Banana Yogurt Ice Cream* Water, *or* 1 cup skim milk	Complex carbohydrate ++ Fiber + Potassium + Calcium + Magnesium +

Day 2

BREAKFAST	Scrambled eggs* 1–2 slices whole wheat toast ½ grapefruit 6 ounces fruit juice	Protein ++ Complex carbohydrate + Vitamin C ++ Fiber +
LUNCH	Tuna Salad Pita Pocket* Crudités* 1 apple, pear, or orange Regular or sparkling mineral water, *or* ½ cup skim milk	Protein ++ Complex carbohydrate ++ Fiber + Vitamin C +
DINNER	Meatless Chili* Cornbread* Tossed green salad with Low-Fat Vinaigrette* Steamed broccoli or zucchini Noodle Kugel* Water, *or* 1 cup skim milk	Protein + Complex carbohydrate ++ Potassium + Fiber ++

Day 3

BREAKFAST	½ cup Noodle Kugel*, *or* 2–3 Buckwheat Pancakes* Apple Puree* 1 additional fruit 6 ounces fruit juice	Complex carbohydrate + + Vitamin C + +
LUNCH	"Chili Dog"* with grated cheese Crudités* 1 apple, pear, or orange Regular or sparkling mineral water	Protein + + Calcium + Fiber + Vitamin C +
DINNER	Ronnie's Broiled Chicken Breasts* Brown rice, *or* Baked Potato with Low-Fat Topping* Steamed broccoli, zucchini, or cauliflower Tossed green salad with Low-Fat Dressing* Baked Apple* Water, *or* 1 cup skim milk	Protein + + Complex carbohydrate + + Fiber + Potassium +

Day 4

BREAKFAST	1 cup Fruity Oatmeal* ½ cup skim milk 6 ounces fruit juice	Complex carbohydrate + + Calcium + Vitamin C +
LUNCH	Chicken Salad* on whole wheat or pita bread Crudités* 1 apple, pear, or orange ½ ounce cheese, *or* ½ cup skim milk Sparkling or regular mineral water	Protein + + Fiber + Potassium + Calcium +
DINNER	Hearty Lentil Soup* Spinach Salad*	Protein + Complex carbohydrate +

Whole wheat bread	Fiber +
Apple Crisp* or Frozen Yogurt*	
Water, *or* 1 cup skim milk	

Day 5

BREAKFAST	2–3 Cottage Cheese Apple Pancakes*	Protein ++

BREAKFAST 2–3 Cottage Cheese
Apple Pancakes*
Apple Puree*
   1 additional fruit
   6 ounces orange juice

Protein ++
Calcium ++
Vitamin C +

LUNCH Spinach Tofu Pita
Pouch*
Crudités*
1 apple, pear, or orange
Bran Muffin*
½ cup skim milk, *or* sparkling
   or regular mineral
   water

Complex carbohydrate ++
Vitamin C ++
Potassium +
Magnesium +

DINNER Broiled Salmon Steak*
Baked Tomatoes*
Baked potato or whole
   wheat pasta
Broccoli Salad*
Rice Pudding* or fresh
   fruit

Protein ++
Calcium +
Vitamin C +
Complex carbohydrate ++
Potassium +

Note: If You Feel You Need More Calories to Sustain You

For Breakfast: Increase cereals by ¼ to ½ cup. Increase toast or pancakes by one slice.

For Lunch: Add more Crudités to each lunch, or one bran muffin, or ½ cup low-fat plain yogurt.

For Dinner: Add Crudités, as much as you desire, to each meal, or one slice whole grain bread.

Snacks: See Chapter 4. You can have one afternoon snack and one after-dinner snack per day. Use suggestions and recipes in this chapter.

General Guidelines for Daily Menus

If you wish to develop your own menus, or get tired of the menus here, use the following guidelines and choose from Martha Rose's recipes in Chapter 11.

2 3- or 4 ounce servings daily of poultry, fish, beans, or tofu (these foods contain protein)
4 ¾-cup servings daily of fruits and/or vegetables (these contain potassium and magnesium)
4 ¾-cup servings daily of high-roughage cereals or grains, *or*
4 slices of whole-grain bread (these contain complex carbohydrates, and fiber)

You can eat as much as you want of the following foods (they contain potassium, sodium, magnesium, and fiber):

bouillon
celery
chicory
Chinese cabbage
all lettuces
parsley
radishes
watercress

Acceptable Commercial Cereals

These cereals contain complex carbohydrates, B complex, and fiber.

oatmeal
shredded wheat
Grape Nuts
Kellogg's Nutri-Grain cereals

Wheatena
Quaker 100% Whole Wheat Cereal
granolas with no extra oils and no sugar
Alpen
Muesli
Bran Chex
Raisin Bran (not sugar-coated)

Competition Diets

Precompetition Meals

The main thing to get into your head is that the steak-and-eggs training breakfast is a thing of the past. It is now common practice to avoid hard-to-digest protein on the day of a big game, and also to avoid fats, oils, and bulky foods or foods that give you gas. The precompetition meal should be small and simple, and should be eaten two hours before competition. Its goals are to provide your muscles with the energy they will need, to prevent hunger during competition, to hydrate the body, and to prevent gastrointestinal upset. Eat high-carbohydrate (complex carbohydrate, that is, 60 to 80 percent) meals, and avoid fats. Drink lots of water, about 1 cup for each 50 pounds of your body weight, and 1 cup for each 15 minutes of strenuous physical activity that you will be engaging in.

Competition-Day Diets

BREAKFAST	¼–½ cup approved cereal of your choice (see list above) ½ cup skim milk 1 fruit 2–3 large glasses water	Complex carbohydrate + Calcium + Vitamin C +
LUNCH	Vegetable Pocket Sandwich* 1 apple 2 Oatmeal Cookies*	Complex carbohydrate + Fiber +

BREAKFAST	2 slices whole wheat toast or whole wheat bagel 2 tablespoons Apple Puree* ½ cup plain low-fat yogurt or cottage cheese 1 fruit 2–3 large glasses water	Complex carbohydrate + Calcium + Vitamin C +
LUNCH	Spaghetti with Cottage Sauce* 1 apple, banana, or orange	Complex carbohydrate + Vitamin C +
BREAKFAST	2 Apple-Raisin Muffins* ½ cup plain low-fat yogurt, cottage cheese, or skim milk 1 banana 2–3 large glasses water	Complex carbohydrate + B complex + Calcium + Potassium +
LUNCH	Baked Potato with Low-Fat Topping* 1 apple, banana, or orange	Complex carbohydrate + Potassium + Vitamin C +
BREAKFAST	Banana Yogurt Smoothie*, or ½ cup Rice Pudding* 1 Bran Muffin*	Calcium + Fiber + Complex carbohydrate +
LUNCH	Tuna Salad* sandwich 2 Oatmeal Cookies* 1 apple, banana, or orange	Protein + Complex carbohydrate + Vitamin C +

Liquid Meals

These are good for before evening competitions.

Banana Yogurt Smoothie* Carob Frappe* Carob Banana Frappe* Peach Buttermilk Shake* Banana Peanut Butter Smoothie*	Potassium + Vitamin C + Fiber +

You can accompany liquid meals with one or two muffins made from the recipes on pages 198–203.

Postcompetition Meals

The purpose of the postcompetition meal is to restore the glycogen burned by your muscles during your exercise, and to replace the fluids, vitamins, minerals, and protein your body has used up. The five postcompetition meals that follow will serve these functions—and taste good, too.

4 ounces fish or poultry
1–2 baked potatoes with low-fat toppings, *or*
   1 cup whole wheat pasta with tomato sauce
   1 cup steamed or raw green, yellow, or orange vegetables
1–2 fresh fruits
   1 pint water (or more as desired)

2 cups beans
2 slices whole-grain bread or cornbread
   1 cup steamed or raw green, yellow, or orange vegetables
Tossed green or spinach salad (optional)
1–2 fresh fruits
   1 pint water (or more as desired)

1 cup beans
1 cup low-fat cottage cheese
   1 cup steamed or raw green, yellow, or orange vegetables
Tossed green or spinach salad (optional)
1–2 fresh fruits
   1 pint water (or more as desired)

1 cup beans
1 cup cooked grains
1 slice whole-grain bread
   1 cup steamed or raw green, yellow, or orange vegetables
Tossed green or spinach salad (optional)
1–2 fresh fruits
   1 pint water (or more as desired)

   1 cup cooked pasta or grains with tomato sauce
   1 cup steamed or raw green, yellow, or orange vegetables
Tofu Sprouts Salad*
1–2 fresh fruits
   1 pint water (or more as desired)

Brown-Bag Breakfasts

If you know you have trouble getting out of bed early enough to eat a decent breakfast before going to school, there is still a way for you to get it, so that you will perform well throughout the day, both in the classroom and on the playing field. You can pack the suggestions below in a bag or lunch box before you go to bed, and grab your breakfast on the way out the door. Then you will have something nutritious to nibble on when that slump comes on at 10:00 A.M. These suggestions will do a lot more for you than the donuts or vending machine cupcakes you used to eat.

1–2 muffins*
½–1 cup plain low-fat yogurt or cottage cheese
hard-boiled egg
2 homemade Granola Bars*
blender drinks* in a thermos
peanut butter on whole wheat bread
Breakfast Cheesecake*
Whole Wheat Bagel* with Low-Fat "Cream Cheese"*

Low-Calorie Diet for Noncompetitors

This diet is for those of you who are starting out on an exercise and diet regimen. It is basically very similar to the *Main Maintenance Diet,* but slightly lower in calories.

Day 1

BREAKFAST   ½ cup approved cereal (see list, page 154)
              ⅓ cup skim milk

½ banana
6 ounces fruit juice

LUNCH   ¾ cup Tuna Salad*
           1 slice whole-grain bread
           Crudités*
           1 apple

DINNER   Ronnie's Broiled Chicken Breast*
           ⅓ cup cooked brown rice
           ½ cup steamed or raw green, yellow, or orange veg-
             etable
           Tossed green salad with Low-Fat Vinaigrette*

Day 2

BREAKFAST 1 soft-boiled egg
           1 slice whole grain toast
           ½ grapefruit

LUNCH   1 cup Gazpacho*, with 2 tablespoons cubed tofu or
             low-fat plain yogurt
           1 slice whole-grain bread •
           Crudités*
           1 pear or orange

DINNER   Poached Filet of Sole with Tomato Puree*
           ½ cup cooked whole wheat pasta
           ½ cup steamed or raw green, yellow, or orange veg- .
             etable
           Tossed green salad with Low-Fat Vinaigrette*

Day 3

BREAKFAST ½ cup low-fat yogurt
           1 slice whole-grain toast
           ¼ cantaloupe

LUNCH   ¾ cup Tofu Sprouts Salad*
           1 slice whole-grain bread
           Crudités*
           ½ apple

DINNER   Curried Cauliflower Soup*
           1 slice whole-grain bread
           Spinach Salad* with Low-Fat Vinaigrette*

Day 4

BREAKFAST   ½ cup Fruity Oatmeal*
                   ¼ cup skim milk
                   6 ounces fruit juice

LUNCH   ¾ cup Low-Fat Egg Salad*
                   1 slice whole wheat bread
                   Crudités*
                   1 peach

DINNER   Stir-Fried Chicken and Vegetables*
                   ⅓ cup cooked bulgur
                   Escarole and Orange Salad*

Day 5

BREAKFAST   1 Whole Wheat Bagel*
                   ¼ cup Low-Fat "Cream Cheese"*
                   ¼ cup Apple Puree*

LUNCH   ¾ cup Chinese Chicken Salad*
                   1 slice whole wheat bread
                   Crudités*
                   ½ cup watermelon balls

DINNER   Puree of Spinach Soup*
                   1 slice whole-grain bread
                   Tossed green salad
                   Banana Yogurt Ice Cream*

Eating in Restaurants

It's possible to stick to the kind of eating we are recommending here and still go to restaurants. You don't have to give up your favorite fast food places. If you did, it would be especially difficult for athletes when you have away games.

At almost all restaurants you can find pasta, rice, baked potatoes, vegetables, chicken, fish, and fruit. Ask for potatoes and grains without butter, and fish and chicken broiled or baked without butter. Eat salads, but ask for the dressing on the side, and use the minimum. Or, even better, ask the waiter for a lemon and season your salad with fresh-squeezed lemon juice (better-tasting by far than the often-rancid bottled salad dressings chain restaurants usually offer. Salad bars are more and more common, and here is where you can really go to town. Pile your plate with vegetables, chick peas, bean salads. Eat cottage cheese and tuna, but stay away from the creamy dressings.

Your best bet for fast food is Mexican, where bean burritos and tacos, with lettuce and tomatoes and the minimum of cheese, will fill your carbohydrate needs without adding lots of fat. Mexican bean burritos or tostadas contain 40 percent fewer calories, one-third the fat, cholesterol, and salt, two times the fiber, six times the vitamin A, and much more thiamine and vitamin C than fast food hamburgers.

The Wendy's chain, and now others, offer a salad bar, so take advantage of that (but don't eat the chili that goes with it more than once a week, as it's full of beef). And at pizza places you can always order small pizzas and remove most of the cheese.

Acceptable Restaurant Meals

Baked potato with low-fat yogurt, cottage cheese, or mustard
Tossed green salad with lemon juice
Fresh fruit
Water

Spaghetti with tomato sauce (without meat preferable, and definitely without sausage)
Tossed green salad with lemon juice
Fresh fruit
Water

Broiled or baked chicken, skin removed
Rice (ask for it without butter)
Steamed green, yellow, or orange vegetable
Tossed green salad with lemon juice
Fresh fruit
Water

Broiled fish (ask for it without butter)
Rice or baked potato with low-fat yogurt, cottage cheese, or mustard
Steamed green, yellow, or orange vegetable
Tossed green salad with lemon juice

Chef's salad with lemon juice
Whole-grain bread (1–2 slices)
Fresh fruit
Water

Spinach salad with chopped eggs (ask for it without bacon), tossed
with lemon juice
Whole-grain bread (1–2 slices)
Fresh fruit
Water

Salad bar: vegetables, beans, cottage cheese, sprouts, chopped egg,
tuna, etc., but toss with vinegar or lemon juice
Whole-grain bread (1–2 slices)
Fresh fruit
Water

Cottage cheese and fruit salad
Whole-grain bread (1–2 slices)
Water

Bean burritos with lettuce and tomato
Tossed green or spinach salad with lemon juice
Fresh fruit
Water

Small pizza (plain) with no extra cheese (remove what cheese you
can)
Tossed green salad with lemon juice
Fresh fruit
Water

CHAPTER 11

How to Eat Well: A Family Diet Plan

Part I: Before You Begin: Getting Organized.

Here are three week's worth of delicious, low-fat meals. The recipes are as easy for the beginner as they are for the seasoned cook. If you teenagers are interested in cooking for yourselves, here is your chance. But no matter who does the cooking, things will go a lot more smoothly throughout the week if you organize your kitchen, making sure to always have certain staples on hand. Feeding yourself well won't be a hassle if you devote one morning or afternoon over the weekend to shopping and precutting vegetables for the next seven days, when school and work take up so much of your time.

Once you've come back from the store with all of your fruits and vegetables, take an hour or so to prepare vegetables. You can work and visit at the same time with family or friends, with the radio or television on for entertainment. It's easy to gossip while chopping vegetables, and working with food can be very relaxing—especially if there's a good movie on the tube to watch while you're doing it. If you get a lot of the busy work done in advance, when the pressure of your hunger is off, you can put meals together in no time, and you'll enjoy them more too.

Vegetable Preparation: Prepare your vegetables for Crudités for the week, and make up baggies for each day, so that you can grab them as you run out the door to catch the bus. See the recipe on page 218 for suggestions and preparation instructions.

Prepare vegetables for soups, salads, and vegetable dishes, and store them separately in sealed plastic bags or containers.

Onions: Chop.

Garlic: Peel cloves and leave whole.

Carrots: Peel.

Green peppers: Chop some, cut others in strips.

Parsley: Wash, dry, and chop.

Lettuce: Separate leaves, wash, dry, and wrap in towels. Refrigerate in sealed plastic bags.

Cucumbers: Chop or slice, according to recipes.

Zucchini: Slice.

Broccoli and cauliflower: Break into florets.

Celery: Slice.

Spinach: Wash, stem, dry, wrap in towels. Refrigerate in sealed plastic bags.

Salad Dressing: Make enough Yogurt Vinaigrette and Tofu Vinaigrette (see recipes) for the week.

Vegetable Stock: Make enough stock for the week and freeze or refrigerate. (You can also use vegetable bouillon or chicken stock for all these recipes).

Grains and Legumes: You can cook grains and beans up to three days ahead of time, so they will be ready when you need them. Both grains and beans also freeze well.

How to Follow a Recipe

Some of you may be beginning cooks: for you, reading a recipe can be like reading a foreign language. To clarify things, here is a glossary of cooking terms and utensils, as well as instructions for preparing vegetables and fruits, and general cooking directions for grains and legumes.

First, though, learn this method for following recipes, so that you and your kitchen will not get completely out of control.

1. Read the recipe from beginning to end first, and make sure you understand the instructions.

2. Prepare and measure out all ingredients *before* you begin cooking, and have them all in reach.

3. Take down all utensils and serving dishes you will need before you begin, and have them within reach.

4. Clean as you go along. Throw away peels and scraps, and clean work surfaces, arranging ingredients on separate plates, or in neat piles. Everything will be much easier if your kitchen doesn't look like a war zone, and you will be grateful for your good habits when it's time to do the dishes.

Cutting Fruits and Vegetables

Onions. First cut in half lengthwise: that is, from the stem end to the other, along one of the lines. Cut the very ends off and remove the skin. Do this near the sink with the cold water running and you won't cry so much. To *chop*, lay one half flat-side-down on your cutting board and cut across the onion in thin stripes, starting at one end and working toward the center. Hold the onion down at the opposite end with your other hand. As the knife nears your fingers, turn the onion around, and, holding onto the side you have already cut to steady the onion, cut again toward the center. Now turn the onion a quarter turn and cut across the slices at a right angle to dice. Repeat for the other half.

If a recipe instructs you to cut an onion in *strips*, place the cut onion on your work surface and cut along the lines of the onion, in the same manner as above, but don't then turn it and cut at a right angle.

For cutting *rings* do not cut the onion in half first. Remove the skin by first cutting the ends off, then cutting a lengthwise slit through the skin one layer deep, all the way around, then removing the skin. Cut the onion crosswise (across the lines) into rings.

Garlic.   First pull off the number of cloves you need from the head. To peel, place the clove on a cutting board and pound it once with the bottom of a jar, or place the flat side of a wide cutting knife over it and lean on the knife. The clove will burst and the skin will pop off. Either put the clove through a press or chop it, holding down the tip of your knife with one hand while you rock the knife up and down with your other. Continue with this motion until the garlic is as finely chopped as you desire.

Green Peppers.   To chop or dice, cut in half lengthwise (from the stem down) and gently remove the stem, seeds, and membranes. Proceed as for onions, cutting into lengthwise strips, then crosswise into dice. For rings, cut the top off, remove seeds and membranes, and cut crosswise.

Tomatoes.   To *peel,* drop the tomatoes into a pot of boiling water. Count to 20, remove from the water, and run under cold water for several seconds. The skin will come away easily. To *seed,* cut in half crosswise (halfway between the stem end and the bottom) and squeeze over a wastebasket or bowl. Don't worry about crushing the tomato, because you are going to cook it anyway. To *chop* tomatoes, cut several strips in one direction, then turn the tomatoes a quarter turn and cut strips in the other direction.

Cucumbers.   When a recipe calls for diced or chopped cucumbers you will probably want to seed them first. This is easy. Cut the cucumber in half lengthwise. The seeds run right down the middle in a neat pattern, and you can scoop them out with a teaspoon, in one movement from one end to the other. To *chop,* cut several narrow lengthwise strips, then cut across these strips at a right angle.

Corn on the Cob.   To remove corn kernels from the cob, stand the cob upright on a plate and run the knife down between the kernels and the cob.

Herbs.   To chop herbs like parsley and basil, place on a cutting board and, using a large knife, chop with quick, rapid strokes, holding the tip down with your spare hand. The herbs will spread out as you chop, but just keep pushing them back to the center. Herbs can also be chopped very efficiently in a food processor.

Slicing Carrots, Zucchini, Celery, or Cucumbers.   When you need a quantity of sliced vegetables, say for a stir-fry, or for Crudités for the week, it's most efficient to line up several, say, carrots, and, using a long, sharp knife, cut several into crosswise slices at one time. Work deliberately and carefully and you won't cut yourself.

Washing Lettuce and Spinach.   Washing leafy vegetables can be very tedious, but there's nothing worse than chomping down on sandy lettuce. If you do a large quantity at a time you won't have to deal with the task every time you want a salad. Separate the leaves and fill the sink or a bowl with cold water. Place in the water, and meanwhile take each individual leaf and run under a cold faucet, rubbing with your thumbs if necessary to make sure all the grit is washed off. Drain on towels and pat dry, or dry in a salad spinner (one of the greatest inventions of the modern kitchen). To store, wrap in towels and place, towel and all, in plastic bags. Seal well and keep in the lower part of your refrigerator.

Broccoli and Cauliflower.   To break into florets, cut cauliflower in half, cut away the stem, and break off the flowers. Cut the tops off the broccoli stems and break into smaller flowers.

Cabbage.   To shred cabbage, cut in quarters and cut away the thick stem. Then cut in thin strips, using a long, sharp knife.

Mushrooms.   If the mushrooms aren't at all sandy, simply cut off the very end of the stem and wipe with a damp cloth. If they are sandy, run briefly under cold water and rub the sand off with your thumbs. Wipe dry with a paper towel or cloth, and trim off the end of the stems. Slice thin.

Apples and Pears. To *dice* or *chop*, make four lengthwise cuts down each side of the core, then slice each piece in one direction, turn a quarter turn and cut again.

Oranges and Grapefruit. To peel and cut away the white pith at the same time, using a very sharp knife cut the skin off in a spiral, starting at the stem end and tilting the knife in slightly. Hold the fruit over a bowl, as it will drip. If you are just peeling to eat or to divide into sections and you don't need to get rid of the pith, quarter the fruit just through the skin with a sharp knife, then peel off the skin in neat quarters.

Cooking Terms

There are just a few cooking terms that need to be defined for the beginner to take the mystery out of cooking. Here they are.

chop or dice: to cut food into small pieces, usually little squares.
mince: to chop very finely, usually using a rocking motion with a large knife, holding down the tip with one hand while you rock your knife-holding hand up and down.
poach: to cook gently in a liquid which is barely simmering on the top of the stove. The liquid is first brought to a simmer, then the food is submerged in it. A very easy and satisfying way to cook fish.
puree: to change the consistency of a food, such as a soup, cooked beans, or vegetables, by blending it in a blender or food processor, mashing it, or putting it through a food mill, so that it becomes smooth or partially smooth. Recipes will specify the extent to which foods should be pureed.
sauté: to cook fairly quickly in a frying pan in a little bit of oil or butter. Here we will try to use nonstick frying pans so that we can use a minimum of oil.
simmer: to cook just at or below the boiling point. The surface is barely bubbling. This is often achieved by bringing to a boil, then reducing the heat to very low.
steam: to cook above boiling water in a lidded pot or steamer. This is a very efficient way to cook vegetables, because their vitamins are not lost in the water as they are when you boil them. To steam, bring a little bit of water to a boil in a lidded pot,

then place your vegetables *above* the water, making sure they aren't submerged, on a steaming trivet, a fold-up steaming basket, a colander, or a Chinese steamer (wooden or aluminum). Eight to 10 minutes is sufficient for most vegetables, like green beans, broccoli, peas, zucchini, and cauliflower. Potatoes, however, take about 20 minutes. Once the vegetables have reached the desired tenderness, remove from the heat and run for a few seconds under cold water to stop the cooking, or serve at once.

stir-fry: to cook quickly, stirring all the time, in a little oil in a frying pan or wok. Here again nonstick skillets are recommended, to reduce the necessary quantity of oil. Don't add the food until the pan is quite hot, or it will just sit and absorb the oil.

General Cooking Directions for Dried Beans

With the exception of lentils and split peas, dried beans (legumes) must be soaked for at least four hours, and preferably overnight, before you cook them. Wash the beans and pick over to make sure there are no little pebbles mixed in with them. Use three parts water per one part beans. Drain the water before you cook, and cook in fresh water. For a very tasty pot of beans, sauté one onion and a few cloves of garlic in your cooking pot before adding the beans. When the onion is soft, add the beans and three parts water and bring to a rolling boil. Make sure the volume of the pot is at least one-third greater than the beans and water, as they will bubble up fairly dramatically. Reduce heat, cover, and simmer one hour (45 minutes for lentils and split peas). Add salt and herbs to taste and continue to simmer, covered, for another hour, or until soft (lentils, split peas, and black-eyed peas take 45 minutes to an hour in all).

General Cooking Instructions for Grains

One cup raw grains feeds four people.

Brown Rice, Barley, Soy Grits.   Use one part grain to two parts water (so for four people, 1 cup either rice, barley, or soy grits with two cups water). Combine the grain and water in a saucepan and bring to a boil. Add ¼ teaspoon salt, reduce heat, cover and simmer 35 minutes, until most of the liquid is absorbed. Remove the lid and cook, uncovered, for 5 to 10 minutes more, or until all the liquid has evaporated.

Millet.   Use 1 part millet to 2½ parts water (so for four people, 1 cup millet with 2½ cups water). Heat 1 teaspoon safflower oil in a saucepan and sauté the millet until it begins to smell toasty and the grains are coated with oil (about 3 to 5 minutes). Add the water and bring to a boil. Add ¼ teaspoon salt, reduce heat, cover, and simmer 35 minutes. Remove the lid and continue to simmer until the liquid is evaporated (up to 10 more minutes).

Wheat Berries, Whole Rye, Triticale.   Use one part grain, three parts water (so for four people, 1 cup grains with 3 cups water). Combine the grains and water and bring to a boil. Add ¼ teaspoon salt, reduce heat, cover, and simmer for 50 minutes. Remove from the heat and pour off any excess liquid.

Bulgur.   Use one part bulgur to two parts water. Place the bulgur in a bowl. Bring the water to a boil and pour over the bulgur. Add ¼ teaspoon salt. Let sit until the water is absorbed and the bulgur soft (about 20 minutes). Pour off excess water and fluff with forks.

Cooking Pasta

Bring a large pot of water to a rolling boil. Add salt and a teaspoon of vegetable or safflower oil and drop in the pasta. Give the pasta a stir with a long-handled spoon so that it doesn't stick together. You only want to cook the pasta until it is cooked through but still firm to the bite—called "al dente"—and this will take anywhere from 4 to 10 minutes, depending on the kind of pasta. Test after 4 minutes and keep testing every minute until it is done. Drain and proceed with your recipe.

Glossary of Ingredients

Some of the ingredients in these menus might be unfamiliar to you. Below is a short glossary. There is nothing very out of the ordinary in the recipes, but you might need to get some of the foods, like the grains, at a natural foods store. The following is by no means a complete list of grains, legumes, etc. It includes only those items that are called for in the recipes in this book.

Grains

Brown Rice: This is unrefined rice, which has a very nutty, wholesome flavor. Both long- and short-grain brown rice is available, and it is easy to find in supermarkets as well as whole foods stores. It takes longer to cook than white rice, but is worth the wait. It is high in B vitamins, is an excellent source of complex carbohydrates, and provides high-quality protein when eaten in combination with dried beans, dairy products, or eggs.

Bulgur is cracked wheat that has been precooked and dried. It's very quick to prepare: all you have to do is pour on boiling water and let it stand for about 20 minutes. Bulgur has a nutty taste and fluffy texture, and has the same nutritional characteristics as brown rice.

Couscous is another precooked cracked-wheat product, made from hard white semolina wheat. It is very light and has a silky texture. All you need to do is pour on warm water to prepare it. It makes a delicious, quick breakfast grain, and is available in imported food stores and many whole foods stores.

Cracked wheat differs from bulgur in that it hasn't been precooked. Makes a great breakfast cereal.

Millet is a delicate, nutty tasting grain that looks like tiny yellow beads. Substitute it for brown rice whenever you want a change. It also makes a nice breakfast grain, and Millet Raisin Pudding is a fine dessert (see page 269).

Rolled or flaked oats: The same thing as oatmeal.

Flaked wheat, rye and triticale: All of these resemble oat flakes, but they are a little stiffer in texture. Triticale is a hybrid grain made from wheat and rye. All of these flakes are made by pressing the whole wheat, rye, or triticale berries. Mix them together with oat flakes for granolas and mixed grain cereals.

Wheat germ: The embryo of the wheat kernel, these tiny flakes are high in oil, protein, and vitamins E and B. Keep refrigerated, as they become rancid quickly.

Legumes

Black beans are black, medium-sized beans with a rich, satisfying flavor. Great for tacos.

Black-eyed peas are medium-sized, oval-shaped, creamy white beans with a black spot on one side. They have a savory, warming flavor.

Garbanzos (or chick peas) are large round beans with a nutty, distinctive taste. Great in salads, soups and blended as a spread.

Kidney Beans are red beans, good in salads and soups.

Lentils have a distinctive, satisfying flavor, and make a delicious soup or salad.

Navy or white beans have a subtle, elegant flavor, and are terrific in soups and salads.

Pinto beans are medium-sized, speckled light brown beans. They are standard in Mexican food. Their flavor is less pronounced than either kidney beans or black beans.

Soybeans are higher in protein than any of the other legumes. Their protein is complete, and they are very economical. Alone they are not very tasty, but with other beans they are good, and roasted they are superb (see page 229). Tofu is made from soybeans.

Soy grits are cracked soybeans, which make a nutritious addition to grain dishes and cereals.

Miscellaneous

Alfalfa sprouts are tiny, delicate sprouts made from alfalfa seeds. Substitute them for lettuce in sandwiches—they don't get soggy—or add to salads any time you wish. They are high in protein, vitamins, and minerals, and easy to find in supermarkets as well as natural foods stores. Other good sprouts are mung bean sprouts, lentil sprouts, and sunflower sprouts.

Arrowroot is basically the same as *cornstarch,* and is used as a thickener. Like cornstarch it must be dissolved in a little liquid before it is used, or it will lump.

Dijon mustard: This French-style mustard, has a sharp, mustardy flavor. It is essential for a good salad dressing, and isn't at all sweet like most American mustards.

Marmite, Vegex, and Savorex are yeast extracts which can be used to flavor soups and tofu preparations. By themselves they are too strong to be appetizing (although English children spread Marmite on their bread), but a little addition of any of these three products will lend a distinctly "meaty" flavor to your dish.

Safflower oil is high in polyunsaturates, and, if made by a reputable company, will not have stabilizers added to it. Store in the refrigerator to prevent rancidity (which you can't always taste).

Sesame tahini is a butter made from ground sesame seeds. It has a marvelous nutty flavor and is a tasty addition to many tofu dishes and salad dressings.

Tamari soy source is a rich, dark soy sauce made by a long, natural fermentation process.

Tofu: This is bean curd, made from soy milk. It is the equivalent of soy cheese. It is a miracle food, very high in protein, low in calories and fat, economical, and extremely versatile. By itself it is bland, with a spongy texture. But like a sponge it will absorb the flavors of whatever it is cooked with, and as it cooks its texture firms up. It can be blended into sauces, makes a low-fat mayonnaiselike vinaigrette, and can be blended up and baked as a quiche. It must be kept in a bowl of water in the refrigerator. Available in supermarkets as well as natural foods stores.

Part II: Menus for Three Weeks, Shopping by the Week, and Helpful Hints

Staples

Before you make your shopping list for the week, you should make a separate list of staples, which you should never be without. These are items which will come up repeatedly in the recipes. Since grains and legumes keep well in tightly sealed jars, you might add your favorite ones to this list, so that you will have them around whenever you want them.

baking powder
baking soda

chicken stock or bouillon cubes

cider vinegar

cornstarch or arrowroot

Dijon mustard

dried fruit (such as raisins, prunes, currants, apricots) for muffins and fruit butters

dry white wine

fresh garlic

fresh ginger (keep in a jar of sherry in the refrigerator)

honey (preferably a light, mild-flavored kind)

Marmite, Savorex, or Vegex (see Glossary of Ingredients, above)

molasses

olive oil

safflower oil

sesame oil

sesame seeds

sesame tahini

sherry

soy sauce

sunflower seeds

unsweetened fruit preserves (homemade or commercial)

vanilla

vegetable bouillon cubes

wine vinegar

Herbs

basil

bay leaves

caraway seeds

cayenne (whole and ground)

cumin seeds
ground cumin
dill seeds
marjoram
oregano
paprika
rosemary
sage
tarragon
thyme

Spices

allspice
cinnamon
ground curry powder
dried ginger
nutmeg
black peppercorns

In Addition

These aren't staples, but this is just to remind you that every week you need to buy vegetables for Crudités, snacks, and soup stocks (see recipe, pg. 242), and fruit for lunches and snacks.

Week-Long Soups and Salads

If you wish, you can double or even triple soup and salad recipes and eat them throughout the week. If you start a great big vegetable soup on a Sunday, say with the vegetables left over from the previous week, you can keep adding to it throughout the following week, and dinner will hardly be a chore at all. By week-long salads I mean those containing beans, grains, and cooked vegetables. These will be good for a few days, so make a quantity over the weekend if you are short on time during the week.

School Lunch in a Jar

School lunches don't always have to consist of sandwiches. Pack leftover salads from dinner in jars, right after dinner, and grab them in the morning as you run out the door.

Breakfast on the Run

Many of the breakfasts, like muffins, blender drinks, even peanut butter sandwiches, can be eaten after you get to school. Once you begin to see that bacon and eggs or cereal with milk aren't the only nutritious breakfasts, you can choose the breakfasts that are easiest for you. If you know you get up too late to prepare or eat a good breakfast at home, prepare it the night before and grab it, along with your lunch, as you rush out to get the bus. This will save you at midmorning, the time you used to be forced to go out and buy a doughnut.

Three Weeks of Menus: Week One

(Asterisk (*) indicates recipe included in following pages.)

Monday

BREAKFAST	1 cup low-fat yogurt 1–2 Bran Muffins* 1 orange	Calcium +++ Complex carbohydrate +++ Potassium + Vitamin C +
LUNCH	Lentil Salad* 1 slice whole grain bread Crudités* 1 apple, pear, or orange	Protein ++ Fiber ++ Potassium + Vitamin C +
DINNER	Chicken-Vegetable Curry* Bulgur Carrot Apple Salad* Banana Yogurt Ice Cream*	Protein +++ Complex carbohydrate ++ Vitamin A + Vitamin C + Calcium +

Tuesday

BREAKFAST   ½ grapefruit   Vitamin C +
                        1–2 soft-boiled eggs   Protein + +
                        Whole-grain toast with   Cholesterol +
                           ¼ teaspoon butter or   Complex carbohydrate + +
                           health margarine

LUNCH   Tabouli* (use last   Complex carbohydrate + +
                        night's bulgur)   Potassium +
                        Crudités*   Vitamin B +
                        2 oatmeal cookies*   Vitamin C +
                        1 fruit   Fiber +

DINNER   Cabbage Apple Soup*   Fiber + +
                        Whole-grain bread   Vitamin B +
                        Warm Potato Salad*
                        Berries with Yogurt*

Wednesday

BREAKFAST   Banana Yogurt   Calcium +
                        Smoothie*   Fiber +
                        1–2 Bran Muffins*
                        (or other muffins of
                        your choice)

LUNCH   Tofu Salad Sandwich*   Protein + + +
                        Crudités*   Potassium + +
                        Fruit   Fiber +
                        1 Granola Bar*

DINNER   Spaghetti with Tofu   Complex carbohydrate + +
                        Tomato Sauce*   Potassium +
                        Whole-grain bread   Vitamin C +
                        Tossed green salad
                        with Low-Fat Dressing*
                        Fruit Ambrosia*

Thursday

BREAKFAST   Fruity Oatmeal*   Complex carbohydrate + +
                        ½ cup skim milk   Fiber +
                        6 ounces fruit juice   Vitamin C +
                                             Calcium + +

LUNCH	Peanut Butter and Honey Sandwich*	Protein +
	Honey Sandwich*	Potassium +
	Crudités*	Fiber +
	Fruit	Sugar +

DINNER	Fish Teriyaki*	Protein +++
	Brown rice*	Complex carbohydrate ++
	Steamed broccoli	Fiber +
	Baked Apple*	Vitamin C +

Friday

BREAKFAST	1 cup granola* or approved cereal (see list in Chapter 10)	Complex carbohydrate ++
		Calcium ++
		Potassium +
		Vitamin C +
	½ cup skim milk	
	1 banana	
	6 ounces orange juice	

LUNCH	Curried Brown Rice Salad*	Complex carbohydrate ++
		Calcium ++
	½ cup plain low-fat yogurt,	Potassium +
	or ½ ounce cheese	Magnesium +
	Crudités*	
	Fruit	

DINNER	Tofu Quiche*	Protein ++
	Steamed Collard Greens with Vinegar*, or	Complex carbohydrate ++
	Steamed green beans or broccoli	Vitamin C +
	Watercress and Mushroom Salad*, or	Potassium +
	Tossed green salad	
	Strawberry Ice*	

Saturday

BREAKFAST	Oatmeal Pancakes*	Complex carbohydrate ++
	Apple Puree*	Vitamin C +
	6 ounces fruit juice	

LUNCH	Corn Chowder*	Complex carbohydrate +++
	Whole-grain bread	Potassium +
	Tomato Salad*	

	2 Oatmeal Cookies* Fruit	Vitamin C +

DINNER	Ronnie's Broiled
	  Chicken Breast*
	Steamed Artichokes
	  with Tofu Vinaigrette*
	Grated Carrot Salad*,
	  or tossed green salad
	Fruit Salad*
		Protein +++
		Complex carbohydrate ++
		Potassium +
		Vitamin C +

Sunday

BREAKFAST	Grapefruit or melon Mushroom Omelette* Whole-grain toast 6 ounces fruit juice	Vitamin C + Protein +++ Complex carbohydrate ++ Fiber ++
LUNCH	Tunafish Salad* Whole-grain bread Crudités* Fruit	Protein ++ Complex carbohydrate ++ Vitamin C + Fiber +
DINNER	Curried Cauliflower Soup* Tossed green salad Whole-grain bread Noodle Kugel*	Complex carbohydrate ++ Potassium + Magnesium +

Three Weeks of Menus: Week Two

Monday

BREAKFAST	2 muffins of your
	  choice*
	½ cup low-fat
	  cottage cheese or plain
	  low-fat yogurt
	6 ounces fruit juice
		Complex carbohydrate ++
		Calcium ++
		Vitamin C +

LUNCH	Low-Fat Egg Salad* sandwich Crudités* 2 Oatmeal Cookies* Fruit	Protein ++ Complex carbohydrate + Vitamin B + Potassium +

| DINNER | Chicken Noodle (or Tofu Noodle) Soup*
Warm Vegetable Salad* (double recipe for tomorrow's lunch)
Whole-grain bread
Poached Bananas* | Protein + +
Complex carbohydrate + +
Potassium + |

Tuesday

BREAKFAST	Whole Wheat Waffles* Apple Puree* or Prune Butter* ½ cup plain low-fat yogurt or cottage cheese 6 ounces fruit juice	Complex carbohydrate + + Vitamin C + Calcium + Protein +
LUNCH	Vegetable Pita Pocket* 2 Oatmeal Cookies* Fruit	Complex carbohydrate + + Vitamin C +
DINNER	Black Beans* (Double recipe for tomorrow's lunch) Cornbread* or corn tortillas Spinach Salad* Oranges with Mint*	Complex carbohydrate + + Protein + Potassium + Vitamin C +

Wednesday

BREAKFAST	Scrambled Eggs* Whole-grain toast ½ grapefruit 6 ounces fruit juice	Protein + + Complex carbohydrate + + Cholesterol + Vitamin C +
LUNCH	Black Bean Burritos* with lettuce and tomatoes Crudités* Fruit	Complex carbohydrate + + Potassium + Vitamin C + Protein +
DINNER	Potato Leek Soup* Tossed green salad Whole-grain bread Breakfast Cheesecake*	Complex carbohydrate + + Potassium + Calcium +

Thursday

BREAKFAST	2 slices whole-grain toast	Complex carbohydrate ++
	Breakfast Cheesecake*	Calcium +
	Fruit of your choice	Vitamin C +
	6 ounces fruit juice	Protein +
LUNCH	Cucumber Cottage Cheese	Calcium +
	Sandwich*	Potassium +
	Crudités*	Complex carbohydrate +
	2 Oatmeal Cookies*	Vitamin C +
	Fruit	
DINNER	Stir-Fried Tofu and Veg-	Protein ++
	etables*	Potassium ++
	Bulgur Pilaf* (make extra	Complex carbohydrate +
	for tomorrow's lunch)	Fiber +
	Oriental Sprouts Salad*	
	Frozen Apple Yogurt*	

Friday

BREAKFAST	Hot Mixed Grains Cereal	Complex carbohydrate ++
	with Fruit*	Calcium ++
	½ cup skim milk	Vitamin C +
	6 ounces fruit juice	
LUNCH	Bulgur Pilaf Salad*	Complex carbohydrate ++
	Crudités*	Potassium +
	½ cup low-fat yogurt or	Calcium ++
	cottage cheese, or ½	Vitamin C +
	ounce cheese	
	Fruit	
DINNER	Broiled Salmon Steak*	Protein +++
	Baked Potato with Low-	Calcium +
	Fat Topping*	Complex carbohydrate ++
	Baked Tomatoes*	Potassium +
	Broccoli Salad*	
	Baked Pears*	

Saturday

BREAKFAST	Apple Smoothie*	Vitamin C ++
	1 –2 Orange Apricot	Fiber +
	Muffins*	Vitamin B +

| LUNCH | Hummus*
Whole-grain bread or pita
Middle Eastern Salad*
Crudités*
Fruit | Complex carbohydrate ++
Potassium +
Vitamin C + |
| DINNER | Homemade Pizza*
Tossed Green Salad*
Banana Yogurt Ice
Cream* | Complex carbohydrate ++
Calcium +
Potassium + |

Sunday

BREAKFAST	Whole Wheat Bagels* Low-Fat "Cream Cheese"* Apple Puree* or Prune Butter* ½ grapefruit 6 ounces fruit juice	Complex carbohydrate ++ Calcium ++ Vitamin C + Fiber +
LUNCH	Mushroom Toasts* Italian-Style Spinach* Mixed Bean Salad* Fruit	Potassium + Vitamin C + Fiber +
DINNER	Minestrone* Whole-grain bread Watercress and Mush- room Salad* Apples with Lime Juice*	Complex carbohydrate ++ Vitamin C + Fiber +

Three Weeks of Menus: Week Three
Monday

| BREAKFAST | 1 cup granola*
½ cup skim milk
1 banana
6 ounces fruit juice | Complex carbohydrate ++
Calcium ++
Potassium +
Vitamin C + |
| LUNCH | Gazpacho*
Whole-grain bread
½ oz. cheese, or ½ cup
low-fat cottage cheese | Complex carbohydrate ++
Calcium ++
Vitamin C + |

	1 Granola Bar* Fruit	
DINNER	Stir-Fried Chicken and Vegetables* Brown rice, bulgur, or millet Spinach and Tangerine Salad* Dried Fruit Compote with Yogurt*	Protein +++ Complex carbohydrate ++ Potassium + Fiber +

Tuesday

BREAKFAST	Scrambled or soft-boiled eggs (2) 1–2 slices whole-grain toast ½ grapefruit 6 ounces fruit juice	Protein ++ Complex carbohydrate + Vitamin C +
LUNCH	Tofu Sprouts Salad* sand- wich Crudités* 2 Oatmeal Cookies* Fruit	Protein + Complex carbohydrate ++ Potassium + Vitamin C +
DINNER	White Bean Soup with Whole-Grain Croutons* Escarole and Orange Salad* or Tossed green salad Brown Rice Pudding*, or Millet Raisin Pudding* (double recipe for tomor- row's breakfast)	Protein + Complex carbohydrate ++ Potassium +

Wednesday

BREAKFAST	Brown Rice Pudding, or Millet Raisin Pudding* ½ cup low-fat yogurt or cottage cheese 6 ounces fruit juice	Complex carbohydrate + Calcium ++ Vitamin C ++

LUNCH	Tuna Salad Pita Pocket*	Protein ++
	Crudités*	Potassium +
	Fruit	Vitamin C +
DINNER	Spinach Lasagne*	Complex carbohydrate +
	Tossed green salad	Potassium +
	Orange Ice*	Vitamin C +

Thursday

BREAKFAST	Banana Peanut Butter Smoothie*	Complex carbohydrate ++
		Protein +
	Bran Muffin*; or whole-grain toast with Apple Puree*	
LUNCH	Cottage, Fruit Salad*	Complex carbohydrate ++
	Crudités*	Potassium +
	Whole-grain bread or crackers	
	2 Granola Bars*	
DINNER	Puree of Spinach Soup*	Complex carbohydrate ++
	Warm Garbanzo Bean Salad* (double recipe for tomorrow's lunch)	Fiber +
		Vitamin C +
	Whole-grain bread	
	Oranges with Figs*	

Friday

BREAKFAST	Couscous with Fruit*	Calcium ++
	½ cup skim milk or plain low-fat yogurt	
	6 ounces fruit juice	
LUNCH	Garbanzo Bean Salad*	Complex carbohydrate ++
	Whole-grain bread or whole wheat pita	Potassium +
	Crudités*	Vitamin C +
	Fruit	
DINNER	Poached Filet of Sole with Tomato Puree*	Protein +++
		Potassium ++

	Steamed New Potatoes with Herbs*	Complex carbohydrate ++ B complex + Vitamin C +
	Steamed zucchini or broccoli	
	Tossed green salad	
	Peach Cobbler*	

Saturday

BREAKFAST	Apple Omelette* Whole-grain toast ½ grapefruit 6 ounces fruit juice	Protein ++ Complex carbohydrate ++ Vitamin C +
LUNCH	Chinese Chicken Salad* Whole-grain bread Crudités* Yogurt Ice Pop*	Protein ++ Complex carbohydrate ++ Potassium + Calcium +
DINNER	Potato Bean Tacos* Salsa Fresca* Steamed zucchini Mexican Salad* Pear Compote*	Complex carbohydrate ++ Protein + Potassium + Fiber +

Sunday

BREAKFAST	Cottage Cheese Pancakes* Apple Puree* 6 ounces fruit juice	Calcium ++ Complex carbohydrate ++ Vitamin C ++
LUNCH	Split Pea Soup* Whole-grain bread Carrot Apple Salad*	Complex carbohydrate ++ Protein + B complex + Fiber + Vitamin C +
DINNER	Cabbage Soup à la Chinoise* Sweet and Sour Shrimp* Brown Rice, bulgur, millet, or couscous Sliced fresh or frozen peaches	Complex carbohydrate ++ Protein ++ Fiber + Vitamin C +

Shopping by the Week

The shopping lists below correspond to the previous menus, for a family of four. Make a checklist and do all of your shopping for the week on the weekend.

Week One

Vegetables and Herbs. Buy enough vegetables for 5 quarts vegetable stock, plus crudités for lunches and snacks for the week (see recipes), plus:

    8 onions
    8 green peppers
    2 bunches parsley
    2 bunches green onions
    3 heads lettuce
    5 cucumbers
    1 bunch radishes
1½ pounds mushrooms
    4 cups bean sprouts or alfalfa sprouts
    3 pounds fresh tomatoes
    4 pounds carrots
    2 heads cauliflower
    2 bunches celery
    1 large red cabbage
    1 zucchini
    3 cups corn kernels (fresh or frozen)
    2 pounds new or russet potatoes
    1 bermuda onion
    1 bunch cilantro
    2 large cans tomatoes (or 3 pounds additional fresh)
    1 bunch fresh basil, if available
    1 bunch broccoli
    2 pounds mustard or collard greens, *or* 1 pound green beans
      or broccoli
    2 bunches watercress (or 1 additional head lettuce)
    3 baking potatoes
    4 artichokes
    fresh herbs if available
    (See also optionals for tossed green salad.)

Fruit.   Buy enough apples, pears, oranges, bananas, etc., for lunches and snacks for everyone in your family for the week, plus:

  8 oranges
16 lemons
24 apples
17 bananas
  5 cups berries (fresh or frozen)
  6 grapefruit (or substitute 1 melon for 2 grapefruit)

Dried Fruit and Nuts

1½ cups currants
1½ cups raisins
  1 cup dates or figs
  2 ounces almonds
  2 ounces shelled walnuts or pecans

Eggs and Dairy Products

  6 quarts plain low-fat yogurt
2½ dozen eggs
  4 ounces Parmesan cheese
  3 quarts skim milk
  ½ pound low-fat cottage cheese
  2 ounces Swiss cheese
  2 ounces other cheese, such as cheddar, Swiss, or jack

Grains, Flours, Legumes, and Pasta

  1 pound whole wheat flour
  ½ pound whole wheat pastry flour
  2 cups bran
  1 cup lentils
  3 cups bulgur
  7 cups oatmeal
  1 cup wheat germ
  2 pounds granola (see recipe if making your own)
  1 pound whole wheat spaghetti
  2 cups brown rice
  ¼ pound flat whole wheat noodles

Tofu, Poultry, and Fish

1¾ pound chicken breasts
4 pounds tofu
1 pound fish filets (add 4 ounces per person extra)
2 cans water-packed tuna

Miscellaneous

1 small can tomato paste
1 ounce unsweetened coconut
5 quarts fruit juice
1 jar natural, unsalted peanut butter
1 quart apple juice

Bread. Buy enough whole-grain bread for sandwiches and
meals for your family for the week. Bread can be frozen, and
buying enough at one time will save you several trips to the
store. Also, buy 10 whole wheat pita breads.

Week Two

Vegetables and Herbs. Buy enough vegetables for 5
quarts vegetable stock, plus crudités for lunches and snacks for
a week (see recipes), plus:

8 onions
6 green peppers
1 bunch celery
2 bunches parsley
3 bunches green onions
1 bermuda onion
1 pound new potatoes
2 bunches broccoli
1 head cauliflower
2½ pounds mushrooms
1 pint cherry tomatoes
1 bunch cilantro
2½ pounds spinach

5 cups bean or alfalfa sprouts
1 bunch fresh mint
15 fresh tomatoes
2 heads lettuce
4 leeks
5 pounds baking potatoes
3 cucumbers
2 bunches radishes
1 bunch dill, if available
5 carrots
1 head Chinese cabbage
4 zucchini (or substitute 1 cup broccoli florets for 1 zuc-chini)
2 bunches watercress
2 large cans tomatoes
1 small can tomatoes
1 green cabbage
1 cup fresh or frozen peas (1 pound fresh, in their pods)

Fruit. Buy enough fresh fruit for lunches and snacks for a week, plus:

Fruit for the muffin recipes of your choice
15 lemons
8 bananas
4 grapefruit (increase if there are more than 4 of you)
6 oranges
12 apples
4 pears
2 limes

Dried Fruit and Nuts

Dried fruit for muffins (see recipe of your choice)
2 cups raisins
1 cup dried apricots
1 ounce shelled walnuts or pecans

Eggs and Dairy Products

5 quarts plain low-fat yogurt
2 quarts skim milk
2 pounds low-fat cottage cheese
2½ dozen eggs
½ pound Parmesan cheese
1 quart buttermilk
6 ounces skim milk mozzarella cheese or gruyère
2 ounces cheddar or Monterey Jack cheese
2 additional ounces swiss cheese
1 stick butter or health margarine
2 additional ounces cheese of your choice

Grains, Flours, Legumes, and Pasta

1 pound rolled oats
4 pounds whole wheat or whole wheat pastry flour
2 pounds dried black beans
½ pound cornmeal
1 pound soybeans
1 pound granola (see recipe if making your own)
1½ pounds bulgur
1 pound unbleached white flour
¼ pound wheat germ
½ pound cracked wheat
¼ pound soy grits
½ pound millet
¼ pound flaked wheat, rye, or triticale
½ pound dried garbanzos, plus 1 additional pound dried
   (or 6 cups canned)
½ pound dried kidney beans (or 2 cups canned)
1 pound dried white beans (or 4 cups canned)
½ pound additional dried beans (or 2 cups canned)
12 ounces flat whole wheat noodles or spaghetti

Tofu, Poultry, and Fish

4½ pounds tofu
½ pound chicken breasts
4 salmon steaks (increase number for more than 4 people)

Miscellaneous

5 quarts fruit juice
1 quart apple juice
2 small cans tomato paste
3 tablespoons active dry yeast (3 packages)

Breads

10 whole wheat pita breads
  6 whole wheat flour tortillas
12 corn tortillas, unless making cornbread to serve with the
    black beans
Whole-grain bread for meals for the week (at least 3 loaves)

Week Three

Vegetables and Herbs.   Buy enough vegetables for Crudités, for 3 quarts vegetable stock (unless you are using bouillon),
plus lunches and snacks for a week (see recipes), plus:

    5 pounds tomatoes
    8 onions
    2 pounds carrots
    4 cucumbers
   10 green peppers
    2 bunches parsley
    1 bunch fresh basil, if available
    5 cups alfalfa or bean sprouts
    1 green cabbage
 2½ pounds zucchini, *or* 1½ pounds zucchini and 1 pound
     broccoli
1½ pounds spinach
    2 pounds mushrooms
    3 bunches green onions
    2 bunches cilantro
    3 heads lettuce
    1 escarole, or 1 additional head lettuce
    2 bunches radishes
    3 large cans tomatoes
    3 packages frozen spinach

1 baking potato
3 pounds new potatoes
Fresh herbs if available, such as dill, thyme, basil
3 jalapeño or serrano chili peppers
2 cups corn kernels
1 sweet red pepper
1 Chinese cabbage
1 cup fresh or frozen peas (1 pound fresh, in pods)
1 bunch celery

Fruit.   Buy enough fruit for lunches and snacks for a week, plus:

10 bananas
12 lemons
1 pound tangerines
4 grapefruit (add if more than 4 people)
8 oranges
12 apples
8 pears
1 pineapple
3 pounds fresh or frozen peaches

Dried Fruit and Nuts

1 cup dried apricots
1 cup prunes
5 cups raisins
½ cup dried pears or peaches
3 ounces figs

Eggs and Dairy Products

4 quarts skim milk
5 quarts plain low-fat yogurt
2 ounces cheese of your choice
3½ pounds low-fat cottage cheese
2½ dozen eggs
10 ounces skim milk mozzarella or farmer cheese
½ pound Parmesan cheese

Grains, Flours, Legumes, and Pasta

2 pounds granola (see recipe if making your own)
1 pound brown rice
½ pound millet
½ pound bulgur
1 pound rolled oats
¼ pound wheat germ
1 pound raw navy beans (or 6 cups canned)
1 pound millet
¼ pound bran
1 pound whole wheat or whole wheat pastry flour
1 pound dried garbanzos (or 4 cups canned)
½ pound couscous
¼ pound corn meal
½ pound black, kidney, or pinto beans (or 3 cups canned)
1 pound split peas
½ pound additional brown rice, bulgur, or millet
12 whole wheat lasagne noodles

Tofu, Poultry, and Fish

1 pound tofu
1 pound chicken breasts
2 cans water-packed tuna
1 pound sole filets
1 pound shrimp

Miscellaneous

1 small can frozen orange juice concentrate
2 quarts apple juice
5 quarts additional fruit juice
1 quart V-8 or tomato juice
1 small can tomato paste
1 jar natural peanut butter
1 quart orange juice

Breads.   Buy enough whole-grain bread for meals for a
week, plus:

12 corn tortillas
6 whole wheat pita breads

Part III: Recipes

Here are the dishes I've been talking about. Martha Rose's recipes will deliver the flavors you are used to, but none of the fats and sugar which make you moody, unsatisfied, overweight, allergic, tired, pimply, unpopular, and depressed. When you begin to eat this food you won't feel like you're on a diet, but in a few weeks time you will begin to feel lighter and happier. The recipes are simple enough for teens or parents to prepare, and everybody in the family will enjoy how this food tastes.

Note: The recipes in this book have been keyed for the various important nutrients that all of us need. Growing, young adolescents should especially use those with three pluses (+++) for calcium, magnesium, B complex, and protein. All of us should strive for low fat and high complex carbohydrates. Some fat is important, but the recipes in this book use a minimal amount. A single plus (+) means that there is a little bit of the indicated nutrient in the recipe; double plus (++) indicates a fair amount; and three pluses (+++) reveals a large amount, but not necessarily the recommended amount for the whole day. You should use these keys to select recipes suited to your needs. For example, if you have trouble falling asleep and have muscle cramps, then the recipes keyed +++ for calcium and magnesium would be appropriate.

Breakfast Dishes and Baked Goods

Grains and Cereals

Fruity Oatmeal

2 cups water
2 cups skim milk (or
   use 4 cups water in all)

Calcium ++
Complex carbohydrate ++
Vitamin C +

    1 teaspoon vanilla extract
    2 cups noninstant oatmeal
    ¼ teaspoon salt (optional)
    3 tablespoons raisins
    ½–1 teaspoon cinnamon
    ½ teaspoon nutmeg
    2 apples, chopped

Combine the water, milk, and vanilla in a saucepan and bring to a boil. Slowly pour in the oatmeal, stirring all the while with a wooden spoon. Add the salt, raisins, cinnamon, nutmeg, and apple, cover, and reduce the heat. Simmer over very low heat for 15 to 20 minutes, until the liquid is absorbed. Serve at once. Top if you wish with a little honey (though you probably won't need it, as the vanilla and raisins with the spices should sweeten this sufficiently) and a little skim milk or plain yogurt. (Serves 4.)

Fruity Oatmeal Made the Night Before

If you are always too rushed in the morning to have a decent breakfast, here is the answer. Before going to bed, place the oatmeal, fruit, and spices in a widemouth thermos. Bring the water and milk to a boil, pour them into the thermos, and seal the thermos tightly. In the morning your breakfast will be ready. If it's not hot enough, simply heat it in a saucepan with a little more water or milk. You can even bring the thermos to school and eat your breakfast during chemistry class.

Mixed Grains Cereal

Mix these grains together and keep on hand for hearty hot cereal.

    1 cup rolled oats
    1 cup cracked wheat
    ½ cup soy grits
    ½ cup cracked millet (this can
      be cracked in a blender)
    1 cup flaked wheat, rye, or triticale
    ¼ cup cornmeal

Complex carbohydrate +++
Calcium +
Magnesium ++
Protein ++

Hot Mixed Grains Cereal with Fruit

2 cups Mixed Grains Cereal	Complex carbohydrate +++
5 cups water, or use half water, half milk	Vitamin C ++
¼ cup raisins	
2 apples, pears, or bananas, chopped	
1 teaspoon cinnamon	
1 teaspoon vanilla	
1 tablespoon honey (optional)	
Salt, to taste	

Bring the water or water and milk to a boil and slowly add the cereal, stirring all the while with a wooden spoon. Add the raisins, fruit, cinnamon, vanilla, honey, and salt to taste, cover, and reduce heat to very low. Simmer 15 to 20 minutes. Remove from the heat and serve, topping with skim milk or yogurt if you wish. (Serves 4.)

Couscous with Fruit

1 cup couscous	Complex carbohydrate ++
2 cups water	Vitamin C ++
½ cup apple juice	
2 teaspoons vanilla	
¼ cup raisins	
1 pear, cored and chopped	
1 apple, cored and chopped	
½–1 teaspoon ground cinnamon, to taste	
½ teaspoon ground nutmeg	
¼ teaspoon allspice	
Plain low-fat yogurt for topping	

Place the couscous in a bowl and pour on the water. Heat the apple juice in a skillet and add the vanilla, raisins, apple, and pear. Cook over medium heat until the fruit begins to soften, about 3 minutes. Add the spices and cook another 3 to 5 minutes.

After about 10 minutes the couscous should be soft. Toss with the fruits over medium heat in the pan until heated through. Serve, topping each serving with a generous spoonful of plain low-fat yogurt if you wish. (Serves 4.)

Homemade Granola

3 cups rolled oats
1½ cups flaked wheat (can
   substitute rolled oats)
1½ cups flaked rye or flaked triticale
   (can substitute rolled oats)
3 cups untoasted wheat germ
1 teaspoon ground nutmeg
2 teaspoons powdered cinnamon
½ cup soy flour
½ cup sesame seeds
1 cup sunflower seeds
1 tablespoon vanilla extract
¼ cup safflower oil
⅓ cup mild-flavored honey (or less;
   try doing without since the raisins
   give a sweet taste)
1 cup raisins

Complex carbohydrate + +
Fiber + +
Vitamin B +

Preheat the oven to 250°. Lightly oil two baking sheets or pans.

Mix together the grains, wheat germ, spices, soy flour, seeds, and the vanilla in a large bowl.

Place the oil and honey together in a pan and heat together over very low heat, just until blended. Pour over the grains and mix together well.

Spread the mixture in the lightly oiled pans and bake in the low oven for about 2 hours, stirring every 15 to 20 minutes to redistribute the grains so that the granola will bake evenly. Switch the pans from one rack to another occasionally. Add raisins during last 20 minutes. (Makes 2½ quarts.)

When the grains are beginning to brown and smell toasty, remove from the oven and cool in the pans. Store in the refrigerator in plastic bags or in a jar. Serve with skim milk or plain low-fat yogurt.

Breads and Spreads

Apple Raisin Muffins

1 cup whole wheat flour	Complex carbohydrate ++
2 teaspoons baking powder	Fiber ++
½ teaspoon salt	Proteins ++
1 teaspoon ground cinnamon	Calcium ++
½ teaspoon allspice	Vitamin C +
1 cup bran	
2 eggs	
¼ cup safflower oil	
4 tablespoons honey (or less)	
1 teaspoon vanilla	
1 cup skim milk or plain low-fat yogurt	
1 cup chopped apple	
½ cup raisins	

Preheat the oven to 375°. Lightly butter muffin tins.

Sift together the flour, baking powder, salt, and spices. Stir in the bran.

Beat together the eggs, safflower oil, honey, vanilla, and milk or yogurt. Quickly stir into the dry ingredients and combine well. Fold in the apple and raisins.

Spoon into the muffin tins and bake 20 minutes in the preheated oven. Cool 10 minutes in the tins, remove from the tins, and serve hot or cooled. These can be frozen. (Makes 15 muffins.)

Banana Nut Muffins or Bread

2 cups whole wheat flour or whole wheat pastry flour	Complex carbohydrate ++
½ teaspoon baking soda	Protein ++
2 teaspoons baking powder	Calcium +
½ teaspoon salt	Magnesium +
1 teaspoon cinnamon	Fiber +
½ teaspoon nutmeg	
¼ cup safflower oil	
¼ cup honey (or less)	
1 teaspoon vanilla	

2 eggs
1⅓ cups mashed ripe banana (about 3
    medium bananas)
½ cup plain low-fat yogurt
½ cup sunflower seeds or chopped walnuts

Preheat the oven to 375°. Butter muffin tins or a 9 × 5-inch bread pan.

Sift together the flour, baking soda, baking powder, salt, and spices.

Beat together the oil, honey, vanilla, and eggs. Stir in the banana and yogurt.

Quickly stir the wet ingredients into the dry, along with the walnuts or sunflower seeds. Spoon into the muffin tins or bread pan. Bake muffins 20 minutes in the preheated oven. Bake bread 30 to 40 minutes, until a tester comes out clean. Cool in the pan or tins for 10 minutes, then remove. These can be frozen. (Makes 16 muffins or 1 loaf.)

Blueberry Rice Muffins

1¼ cups whole wheat flour
2 teaspoons baking powder
½ teaspoon salt
3 tablespoons honey (use less if
    you can)
¼ cup safflower oil
2 eggs
⅔ cup skim milk or plain low-fat yogurt
1 cup blueberries
1 cup cooked brown rice (may
    substitute other grains)

Complex carbohydrate ++
Protein ++
Calcium ++
Vitamin C +

Preheat the oven to 400°. Lightly butter muffin tins.

Sift together the flour, baking powder, and salt.

Beat together the honey, oil, eggs, and milk. Stir into the dry ingredients. Fold in the blueberries and brown rice or other cooked grains.

Spoon the batter into the prepared muffin tins and bake 20 minutes in the preheated oven. Cool for 10 minutes in the tins, then remove from the tins and serve warm or cooled. These can be frozen. (Makes 15 muffins.)

Bran Muffins

1 cup whole wheat flour	Complex carbohydrate ++
1 cup bran	Fiber ++
1 teaspoon cinnamon	Protein ++
½ teaspoon nutmeg	Calcium ++
½ teaspoon salt	
1 tablespoon baking powder	
2 eggs	
3 tablespoons safflower oil	
2 tablespoons honey, *or* 1 tablespoon molasses, 1 tablespoon honey	
1 cup plain low-fat yogurt	

Preheat oven to 400°. Oil muffin tins.

Mix together the flour, bran, cinnamon, nutmeg, salt, and baking powder.

In a separate bowl beat together the eggs, safflower oil, honey and/or molasses, and the yogurt.

Quickly stir the dry ingredients into the wet ingredients (or vice versa). Do not overbeat (don't worry if there are a few lumps). Spoon into muffin tins, filling two-thirds full with the batter.

Bake 20 minutes in the preheated oven, or until firm and brown. Remove from the heat, let sit in the tins for 5 to 10 minutes, then remove from the tins (run a knife around the edges if they stick) and cool on racks, or serve warm. Store in a plastic bag.

These can be frozen. To thaw, heat through for 15 minutes at 350°.

(Makes 12 to 15 muffins.)

Cornbread or Cornbread Muffins

1 cup stone-ground corn meal	Complex carbohydrate ++
½ cup whole wheat flour	Fiber +
¾ teaspoon salt	Calcium ++
1 tablespoon baking powder	Protein ++
½ teaspoon baking soda	
1 cup plain low-fat yogurt	
½ cup skim milk	

1 tablespoon honey (or a teaspoon would do)
2 eggs
1 tablespoon safflower oil
1 tablespoon butter or margarine

Preheat the oven to 425°.

Sift together the corn meal, whole wheat flour, salt, baking powder, and baking soda in a bowl. In a separate bowl beat together the yogurt, milk, honey, eggs, and safflower oil.

Place the butter or margarine in a 9 × 9-inch baking pan or a 9-inch cast-iron skillet and place in the oven for a few minutes, until the butter melts and begins to sizzle. Remove from the oven and brush the butter all over the sides and bottom of the pan. Pour whatever butter remains into the liquid mixture.

Fold the wet ingredients into the flour mixture. Do this quickly, without overworking the batter. Don't worry if there are a few lumps.

Pour the batter into the prepared baking dish and place in the preheated oven. Bake 30 to 35 minutes, until the top browns and a tester when inserted comes out clean.

Note: You can also make muffins using the same recipe. Bake 20 minutes. (Makes 12 muffins.)

Cranberry Muffins

¾ cup whole wheat flour
¾ cup rye flour
½ cup stone-ground yellow corn meal
2 teaspoons baking powder
¼ teaspoon salt
¼ cup bran
2 eggs
¼ cup safflower oil
2 tablespoons honey
1½ cups buttermilk
1¼ cups coarsely chopped cranberries

Complex carbohydrate ++
Fiber ++
Protein ++
Calcium ++

Preheat the oven to 400°. Lightly butter muffin tins.

Sift together the flours, corn meal, baking powder, and salt. Stir in the bran.

Beat together the eggs, safflower oil, honey, and buttermilk. Stir in the cranberries. Quickly stir into the dry ingredients.

Spoon the batter into muffin tins and bake 20 to 25 minutes. (Makes 14 muffins.)

Orange Apricot Muffins

⅔ cup chopped dried apricots
1 cup whole wheat flour
½ cup unbleached white flour
2 teaspoons baking powder
½ teaspoon salt
½ cup wheat germ
2 oranges
½ cup skim milk
2 eggs
2 tablespoons honey (or less)
2 tablespoons safflower oil

Complex carbohydrate ++
Fiber ++
Vitamin C +
Calcium ++
Protein ++

Place the chopped dried apricots in a bowl and pour boiling water on them to cover. Let sit for 10 minutes, while you prepare the batter, then drain and squeeze dry between paper towels.

Preheat the oven to 375°. Oil or butter your muffin tins.

Squeeze enough juice from the oranges to make ½ cup. Combine with the milk. Take one of the squeezed orange rinds and chop coarsely. Place in a blender with the milk, eggs, honey, and safflower oil and blend until peel is finely chopped.

Sift together the dry ingredients. Add the wet ingredients and quickly mix together. Fold in the chopped apricots.

Spoon the batter into the prepared muffin tins and bake 20 minutes, or until lightly brown and a tester comes out clean. Cool 10 minutes in the tin, then remove and serve. These can be frozen. (Makes 15 to 18 muffins.)

Sweet Potato Muffins

1 cup unbleached white flour   Complex carbohydrate ++

1 cup whole wheat pastry flour
2 teaspoons baking powder
½ teaspoon baking soda
1 teaspoon cinnamon
¼ teaspoon nutmeg
¼ teaspoon salt
¼ cup safflower oil
⅓ cup honey
3 eggs
1⅓ cups cooked mashed
  sweet potatoes
½ cup skim milk or plain
  low-fat yogurt

Fat +
Protein ++
Cholesterol +
Potassium +
Calcium +

Preheat the oven to 400°. Lightly butter muffin tins.

Sift together the flours, baking powder, baking soda, spices, and salt.

Beat together the oil, honey, eggs, sweet potatoes, and milk or yogurt. Stir into the dry ingredients.

Spoon into the prepared muffin tins and bake for 25 to 30 minutes in the preheated oven, until beginning to brown. Cool 10 minutes in the pans, then remove from the tins and cool on a rack. Serve warm or cooled. These can be frozen. (Makes 16 to 18 muffins.)

Whole Wheat Bagels

It's not difficult to find whole wheat bagels in most bagel stores, but if you want to make them yourself, you'll find this recipe very easy.

For the Dough:
1½ cups lukewarm water
2 tablespoons active dry yeast
1 teaspoon honey
1 scant tablespoon salt
3 cups whole wheat flour or
  whole wheat pastry flour

Complex carbohydrate ++
Protein ++

1–1½ cups unbleached white flour
   (up to ½ cup additional for
      kneading)

For the boiling:
   2½ quarts boiling water
   1 tablespoon sugar

For the topping:
   1 egg white
   1 tablespoon water
   1–2 tablespoons sesame seeds or
      poppy seeds

Dissolve the yeast in the water and add the honey. Let stand about three minutes. Stir in the salt and two cups of the whole wheat flour. Beat vigorously with a whisk or at medium speed in a mixer for about 5 minutes. Fold in the remaining whole wheat flour and a cup of the unbleached white flour. Now knead the dough with a dough hook or by hand, either right in the bowl or on a floured surface, adding unbleached flour as necessary. The dough will be sticky at first but should stiffen up after 5 minutes of kneading. Knead for about 8 minutes with a dough hook, 10 minutes by hand, until stiff and elastic.

Oil your bowl. Shape the dough into a ball and place in the bowl seam-side-up first, then turn it so that it lies seam-side-down. Cover and allow to rise in a warm spot until doubled in size, about 1 to 1½ hours.

Bring the 2½ quarts water to a boil in a large pot. Turn down the heat to simmer. Meanwhile punch down the dough and divide into 8 to 10 equal pieces. Form these into balls and let them sit about 4 minutes. Then flatten each ball slightly and make a hole in the center by sticking your thumb through and spreading the center apart with your fingers. Stretch the hole out a little bigger than you want it to look when the bagels are done, because as they rise the holes will shrink. Place on a floured surface and cover with a towel or wax paper. Let rise ten minutes while you preheat the oven to 450°.

Now you will boil the bagels to get the beginning of your

sleek, chewy crust. Have the water gently boiling and add the sugar (this gives them their shine). Using a wide spatula or skimmer gently lift the bagels, in batches of two or three, and lower into the boiling water. After 25 seconds flip the bagels over so that they boil on both sides. Leave 25 more seconds, carefully lift from the water, and drain on a towel. Repeat with all the bagels.

Oil a couple of baking sheets and sprinkle with corn meal. Beat together the egg whites and water and gently brush the bagels. Sprinkle with the poppy or sesame seeds and transfer to the baking sheets. Bake in the hot oven for 30 minutes, switching the position of the sheets halfway through the baking. Ten minutes before the bagels are done, flip them over so that the bottom side won't brown too much. Bagels are done when dark brown and shiny.

Cool on a rack. (Makes 8 to 10 bagels.)

Low-Fat "Cream Cheese"

1 cup low-fat cottage cheese	Calcium +++
	Protein ++
¼ cup plain low-fat yogurt	

Blend together the cottage cheese and yogurt in a food processor or electric mixer until smooth. Use as a spread instead of cream cheese. (Makes 1¼ cups.)

Apple Sauce or Puree

6 tart apples, cored and chopped	Vitamin C ++
½ cup water or apple juice	
1 tablespoon honey (or even none at all)	
½–1 teaspoon cinnamon	
¼–½ teaspoon nutmeg	
Juice of 1 lemon	

Combine all the ingredients in a saucepan and simmer together over low heat for 45 minutes to an hour, stirring from time to time with a wooden spoon, until the mixture is thoroughly softened. Mash to puree with the back of the spoon. Eat warm or chilled, plain, with yogurt, or as a spread on toast. This also makes a nice snack. (Serves 4 to 6.)

Prune Butter

1 cup pitted prunes	Calcium ++
Boiling water to cover	Fiber ++
½ cup plain low-fat yogurt	

Place the prunes in a bowl and pour on boiling water to cover. Let sit overnight or for several hours. Drain, retaining a little bit of the liquid. Puree in a food processor or blender, using a little of the soaking liquid, if necessary, to moisten. Stir in the optional yogurt. Use as a spread for toast. (Makes 1 cup.)

Egg Dishes, Pancakes, and a Breakfast Cheesecake

Scrambled Eggs

4 whole eggs	Protein +++
4 egg whites	
Pinch of salt	
Freshly ground pepper to taste	
1 teaspoon butter	
(Optional: for a different taste, try adding a sprinkle of dried basil)	

Beat together the whole eggs and the egg whites. Add a pinch of salt and freshly ground pepper to taste.

Melt the butter in a nonstick skillet over medium-low heat. Add the eggs and stir over the medium-low flame until they reach the desired consistency. Serve at once, with whole grain toast. (Serves 4.)

Apple Omelette

2 tart apples, such as Granny Smith, cored and sliced	Protein ++
	Calcium +
1 teaspoon safflower oil	Vitamin C +
4 eggs	

    4 egg whites
¼ teaspoon ground ginger (optional)
    2 tablespoons grated gruyère or ched-
        dar cheese

Heat the broiler.

Heat the safflower oil in a large, nonstick frying pan and sauté the apples over medium heat until just tender, about 5 minutes. Spread evenly over the bottom of the pan.

Beat together the eggs, egg whites, and optional ginger in a bowl. Heat the pan over a medium-high flame and pour in the eggs. Shake gently over the heat, and lift the edges of the eggs, tilting the pan so the eggs will run underneath. When the eggs are almost cooked through (after about 3 minutes) and there is still a runny layer on the top, sprinkle with the cheese and place the pan under the broiler. Cook under the broiler for 2 to 3 minutes, watching closely, until the top browns slightly. Remove from the heat and serve, cutting the flat omelette in wedges. (Serves 4.)

Mushroom Omelette

    1 tablespoon safflower oil
    2 cups sliced mushrooms
1–2 cloves garlic, to taste, minced
        or put through a press
¼ teaspoon thyme
½ teaspoon soy sauce
Freshly ground pepper to taste
    2 tablespoons chopped fresh
        parsley
    4 eggs
    6 egg whites

Protein ++
Complex carbohydrate +
Vitamin A +

Heat the safflower oil in a nonstick omelette pan and sauté the mushrooms with the garlic. When the mushrooms begin to be tender, add the thyme and soy sauce. Continue to sauté over medium heat for about 5 minutes, until tender and aromatic. Add freshly ground pepper and the parsley, and transfer to a bowl or plate.

Beat the eggs and egg whites together in a bowl. Heat the

omelette pan and pour in the eggs. Swirl the pan to coat the surface evenly, and when a layer has cooked on the bottom, lift the edges with your spatula and tilt the pan so the eggs can run underneath. Spread the mushrooms down the center of the omelette and gently fold over. Cook another minute or so, and turn out onto a large plate or platter. Divide into four portions and serve.

Note: This can also be made as four individual omelettes.

Buckwheat Pancakes

2 eggs, separated	Complex carbohydrate ++
1 tablespoon honey (or just a smidgen)	Protein ++
	Calcium ++
1 cup skim milk	Fiber +
1 tablespoon safflower oil	
¾ cup sifted whole wheat pastry flour	
¾ cup sifted buckwheat flour	
¼ teaspoon salt	
1 teaspoon baking powder	

Beat together the egg yolks, honey, milk, and safflower oil.

Sift together the flours, salt, and baking powder. Stir into the liquid ingredients.

Beat the egg whites until stiff but not dry. Gently fold into the batter.

Heat a large, heavy, preferably nonstick frying pan over a medium-high flame and brush with a small amount of oil or butter. Drop the batter on by heaping tablespoons, or small ladlefuls, so that the pancakes are not too big. Cook on the first side until bubbles break through, then turn and cook until golden brown on the other side. Serve at once, with one of the fruit purees on pages 205–206, and plain low-fat yogurt or cottage cheese. (Makes 18 pancakes.)

Whole Wheat Buttermilk Waffles

2 cups buttermilk	Calcium ++
2 eggs, separated	Protein +++
1 tablespoon honey (try it with less)	
2 tablespoons safflower oil	

2 cups whole wheat flour or whole
    wheat pastry flour
2 teaspoons baking powder
¼ teaspoon salt
    Optional:
1 cup sliced bananas, *or*
1 cup blueberries, *or*
1 cup sliced strawberries, *or*
1 cup chopped apples, pears, or peaches

Blend together the buttermilk, egg yolks, honey, and safflower oil in a food processor or electric mixer. Add the dry
ingredients and combine well, but don't overbeat. Beat the egg
whites until stiff but not dry, and fold into the batter. Stir in the
optional fruit.

Heat your waffle iron until the indicator shows it is ready for
use. Cover the surface about two-thirds full and cook until the
iron stops steaming (about 5 minutes). Waffles should be golden
and crisp.

Serve with Apple Puree (page 205), Prune Butter (page
206), or blended fruit, and plain low-fat yogurt. (Serves 4 to 6.)

Note: These can be frozen and reheated in a toaster or warm
oven.

Cottage Cheese Apple Pancakes

4 eggs
½ cup skim milk
1 cup low-fat cottage cheese
½ teaspoon vanilla
1–2 tablespoons honey, to taste (but try to
    do without, eventually)
½ cup whole wheat flour
¼ cup wheat germ
1 teaspoon cinnamon (or more, to
    taste)
1 cup chopped apple
2 teaspoons safflower oil for the skillet
    (more as needed)

Complex carbohydrate ++
Protein +++
Calcium ++

Blend together the eggs, milk, cottage cheese, vanilla, and
honey.

Stir together the flour, wheat germ, and cinnamon. Stir this into the wet mixture. Stir in the apple.

Heat a nonstick skillet over a medium-high flame. Brush with 2 teaspoons safflower oil and drop the batter in by heaping spoonfuls (about 3 tablespoonfuls; using a ladle makes this easier). The skillet must be very hot. Cook on one side until bubbles break through, then carefully turn and cook until brown on the other side. Keep warm in a low oven. Serve topped with plain low-fat yogurt or Apple Puree (page 205), or a little honey or maple syrup. (Serves 4.)

Oatmeal Pancakes

¾ cup rolled oats
Boiling water to cover oats
  1 cup skim milk
  1 tablespoon safflower oil
  2 eggs
  1 tablespoon honey (or just
    a drop, or even leave it
    out!)
½ teaspoon vanilla
Pinch of salt
¾ cup whole wheat flour
  1 teaspoon baking powder
  2 teaspoons safflower oil
    for the skillet

Complex carbohydrate + +
Calcium + +
Protein + +
Vitamin B +

Place the rolled oats in a bowl and pour on just enough boiling water to cover. Let sit 10 minutes.

Beat together the milk, oil, eggs, honey, and vanilla. Stir in the oats. Mix together the salt, flour, and baking powder and stir into the wet ingredients. Combine well.

Heat a nonstick skillet over medium-high heat and brush with 2 teaspoons safflower oil. Drop the pancakes in by heaping spoonfuls (about 3 tablespoons) and cook until bubbles break through. Skillet should be hot. Turn and cook on the other side until brown. Keep warm in a low oven.

Serve, topping with plain low-fat yogurt and Apple Puree (page 205). These can be reheated in a medium oven, and will have a satisfying, crisp texture. (Serves 4.)

Breakfast Cheesecake

Try this for a real breakfast treat.

For the crust:
 ½ cup granola
 2 tablespoons melted butter
 1 tablespoon honey (or less)

Complex carbohydrate + +
Fat +
Protein + +
Calcium + +

For the filling:
 4 eggs
 2 cups cottage cheese
 ½ cup yogurt
 2 teaspoons vanilla
 2 tablespoons lemon juice
 ¼ cup honey (or a little less)
 ½ teaspoon cinnamon
 2 teaspoons cornstarch
Freshly ground nutmeg to taste (optional)

For the topping:
1½ plain low-fat yogurt
 1 teaspoon vanilla
 2 tablespoons honey

Preheat the oven to 350°. Lightly butter a 1- or 1½-quart rectangular baking dish. Combine the ingredients for the crust and spread evenly in the baking dish.

Blend together the ingredients for the filling in a food processor or a blender. Pour into the baking dish and bake in the preheated oven for 30 minutes.

Stir together the ingredients for the topping and gently spread over the top of the cheesecake. Continue to bake another 10 to 15 minutes or until firm. Cool for 1 hour, then chill. (Serves 6.)

Low-Fat Blender Drinks

Banana Smoothie

1 cup skim milk, *or* ½
 cup orange juice
 mixed with ½ cup
 skim milk

Calcium + +
Potassium +

1 banana
½ teaspoon vanilla
Nutmeg to taste
2–3 ice cubes

Blend all the ingredients together in a blender until smooth and frothy.

Banana Peanut Butter Smoothie

Add 1 tablespoon natural peanut butter to the recipe above.

Carob Frappe 1 serving

1 cup skim milk　　　　　Calcium ++
1 tablespoon carob powder
1 teaspoon vanilla
1 teaspoon molasses
3 ice cubes

Blend all the ingredients together in a blender until smooth and frothy.

Carob Banana Frappe

Add ½ banana (or ½ frozen banana) to the recipe above.

Banana Strawberry Smoothie

1 cup skim milk or plain low-fat yogurt, *or*　　　Protein +
½ cup orange juice mixed with ½ cup　　　　　Calcium ++
　　milk or yogurt　　　　　　　　　　　　Vitamin C ++
1 cup fresh or frozen hulled strawberries　　　Potassium +
½ banana
½ teaspoon vanilla
Nutmeg or cinnamon to taste (optional)
3 ice cubes

Blend all the ingredients together in a blender until smooth and frothy.

Pineapple Banana Mint Smoothie

½ cup orange juice　　　　Vitamin C ++
½ cup plain low-fat yogurt　　Calcium ++
½ banana　　　　　　　　Potassium +

1 cup chopped fresh ripe pineapple
1 tablespoon chopped fresh mint
3 ice cubes

Blend all the ingredients in a blender until smooth and frothy.

Fruit and Sprout Smoothie

1 cup orange or apple juice	Vitamin C ++
½ cup plain low-fat yogurt	Calcium ++
2 tablespoons fresh mint	Fiber +
½ banana	Protein +
½ cup alfalfa sprouts	
3 ice cubes	

Blend all the ingredients together in a blender until smooth and frothy.

Carrot Apple Drink

½ cup plain low-fat yogurt	Calcium ++
1 large carrot, chopped	Protein +
1 tablespoon wheat germ or granola	Complex carbohydrate +
½ cup apple juice or orange juice	Fiber +
½ teaspoon cinnamon	
½ apple, cored and chopped	
2 figs or pitted prunes	
3 ice cubes	

Blend all the ingredients together in a blender until smooth and frothy.

Apple Smoothie

1 cup plain low-fat yogurt, or	Calcium ++
½ cup apple juice mixed with ½ cup plain low-fat yogurt	Protein +
	Vitamin C +
1 apple, cored and chopped	
½ teaspoon cinnamon	
¼ teaspoon nutmeg	
½ teaspoon vanilla	
½ banana	

½ teaspoon honey
3 ice cubes

Blend all the ingredients together in a blender until smooth
and frothy.

Peach Buttermilk Smoothie

1 cup buttermilk   Calcium + +
2 fresh peaches, pitted   Vitamin C + +
½ banana
1 teaspoon vanilla
¼ teaspoon cinnamon
Nutmeg to taste
3 ice cubes

Blend all the ingredients together in a blender until smooth
and frothy.

Lunch Dishes
Sandwiches and Spreads
"Chili Dogs"

4 whole wheat hamburger or hot dog buns   Protein + + +
    (available in health food stores)   Calcium + +
2 cups Meatless Chili (see page 252)   Fiber +
¼ cup grated cheddar cheese
Shredded lettuce or alfalfa sprouts

Top each bun with ½ cup Meatless Chili, a tablespoon of
grated cheese, and shredded lettuce or alfalfa sprouts to taste.
Wrap tightly in plastic if carrying to school (these tend to drip).
(Serves 4.)

Chicken Salad

2 cups diced cooked chicken breast   Protein + + +
1 green pepper, chopped   Potassium +
1 small onion, chopped
½ cup chopped cucumber or celery

1 cup Yogurt Vinaigrette, Curried Yogurt
  Vinaigrette, or Tofu Vinaigrette (pages
  219–220).
1 teaspoon freshly grated ginger (optional)
½ teaspoon soy sauce (optional)

Toss together the chicken, chopped vegetables, and dressing
of your choice. Add fresh ginger and soy sauce as desired. Serve
at once, or chill and serve. This is good for sandwiches too. Try
filling pita breads with it for school lunches. (Serves 4.)
Note: You can substitute diced tofu for the chicken.

Peanut Butter and Honey Sandwich

1 tablespoon unsalted, natural peanut butter (no stabilizers, sugar, or fats added)	Complex carbohydrate ++ Protein + Fat +
1 teaspoon honey	
2 slices whole-grain bread	
Optional: ½ banana, sliced	

Spread the peanut butter on the bread, top with honey and
optional banana. This will really get you through the afternoon.
It makes a good breakfast too.

Tofu Salad Sandwich

½ pound tofu	Protein +++
Soy sauce to taste	Vitamin C +
½ teaspoon freshly grated ginger (or ¼ teaspoon powdered)	Complex carbohydrate ++
½–1 teaspoon curry powder, to taste	
1 small green pepper, minced	
1 carrot, grated	
½ cup alfalfa, mung bean, or lentil sprouts	
2–3 tablespoons chopped fresh coriander (optional)	
1 stalk celery, minced	
½ cup Tofu Vinaigrette (page 219)	
Whole-grain bread or whole wheat pita bread	

Mash together the tofu, soy sauce, ginger, and curry powder. Toss with the green pepper, carrot, sprouts, fresh coriander, celery, and Tofu Vinaigrette. Adjust seasonings, adding lemon juice, mustard, soy sauce, or curry powder if you wish. Make sandwiches on whole-grain bread, or fill whole wheat pita bread with the mixture. You can also eat as a salad.

This will last for about 3 days in the refrigerator. (Serves 4.)

Vegetable Pita Pockets

4 whole wheat pita breads, cut in half	Complex carbohydrate + +
2 cups Marinated Vegetables (see page 220)	Potassium + +
	Calcium + +
1 cup cubed or grated low-fat mozzarella, farmer cheese, or gruyère	Fiber +

Cut the pitas in half and open up the pockets. Toss together the vegetables and cheese, and stuff the pockets with the mixture. Wrap tightly in plastic and carry to school, or eat right away.

Note: This can also be heated in a medium oven, until the cheese melts. (Serves 4.)

Spinach and Tofu Pita Sandwiches

6 ounces spinach, washed, stemmed and dried	Complex carbohydrate + +
¾ pound tofu	Potassium +
1–2 teaspoons soy sauce, to taste	Calcium + +
1 cup Tofu Vinaigrette (page 219)	Protein + +
4–6 large whole wheat pita breads, cut in half	
½ cup alfalfa sprouts (optional)	
Sliced tomatoes (optional)	

Place the spinach, tofu, soy sauce, and Tofu Vinaigrette in a food processor and chop and blend together, using the pulse action of your processor. The spinach should be finely chopped but not pureed. Stuff the pita pouches with this mixture, and add sliced tomatoes and sprouts if you wish. (Serves 4 to 6.)

Tuna Salad Pita Pockets

1 can water-packed tunafish
½ cup chopped green pepper,
  cucumber, or celery
¼ cup minced onion
½ cup plain low-fat yogurt or Tofu
  Vinaigrette (page 219)
Lettuce or alfalfa sprouts
2 whole wheat pita breads

Complex carbohydrate +
Protein +++
Potassium +

Drain the tunafish and mix with the chopped vegetables and the yogurt or Tofu Vinaigrette. Cut a slit in the end of each pita bread and line with lettuce leaves or alfalfa sprouts, then stuff with the tuna mixture. Wrap in plastic wrap. (Serves 2.)

Cucumber Cottage Cheese Spread

1½ cups plain low-fat cottage cheese
½ cup minced cucumber
1 tablespoon chopped fresh dill or
  parsley
1 teaspoon dill seeds or cumin seeds
  (optional)
Juice of ½ lemon
Freshly ground pepper to taste

Calcium ++
Potassium +
Magnesium +

Combine all the ingredients and mix thoroughly. Use as a spread for sandwiches on whole-grain bread or as a filling for whole wheat pita breads, or eat as a salad. (Makes 2 cups.)

Hummus (Middle Eastern Garbanzo Bean Puree)

2 cups cooked garbanzo
  beans (may use canned)
2 large cloves garlic
¼–⅓ cup lemon juice, to taste
¼–½ teaspoon ground cumin, to taste
½ cup plain low-fat yogurt
3 tablespoons sesame tahini
Salt to taste

Protein ++
Calcium +
Complex carbohydrate ++

Puree all the ingredients together in a food processor or blender until smooth. Refrigerate in a covered container. Use as a spread on whole-grain bread or pita bread, or as a dip for vegetables. This will keep for 5 days in the refrigerator. (Makes 2½ cups.)

Salads and Dressings

Crudités

If you always have cut up vegetables on hand you will always have something you can munch on, and you won't have to exercise any will power, because you can munch on as many vegetables as you want. Have a jar of mustard around, or one of the dips or low-fat dressings on pages 219–220, to pep them up a bit. Keep assorted prepared crudités in plastic bags, and carry them to school with you. They will provide you with potassium, sodium, magnesium, and other minerals, as well as fiber and Vitamin A.

Suggested Vegetables:
Carrots, peeled and cut in sticks or rounds
Celery, leaves trimmed, cut in 3-inch sticks
Cucumbers, cut in spears or rounds
Cauliflower, cut into florets
Broccoli, steamed briefly and cut in florets
Mushroom caps, wiped clean

Tossed Green Salad

¾ pound lettuce, any kind, washed well and dried	Complex carbohydrate ++
	Potassium ++
½ cucumber, sliced thin	Protein +
4 radishes, sliced thin	Vitamins B and C +
4 mushrooms, sliced thin	
3 green onions, sliced	
½–1 cup bean sprouts	
2 tomatoes, cut in wedges	
½ green pepper, cut in strips	

Low-Fat Vinaigrette of your choice (see below)
Optional
    cooked garbanzos or other beans
    cubed tofu

leftover cooked grains, such as rice, bulgur, wheatberries
leftover or freshly steamed vegetables, such as cauliflower, broccoli, zucchini, beets, green beans, corn, peas

Toss together all the ingredients with the dressing of your choice and serve at once. (Serves 4 to 6.)

Low-Fat Vinaigrette 1: Yogurt Vinaigrette

Juice of ½ lemon
  3 tablespoons wine or cider vineger
  1 teaspoon Dijon mustard
  1 clove garlic, minced or put through a press
    (optional)
¼ teaspoon tarragon
¼ teaspoon marjoram
Freshly ground pepper to taste
¾ cup plain low-fat yogurt

Potassium ++
Calcium ++
Minerals +

Mix together the lemon juice, vinegar, mustard, garlic, herbs, and pepper. Whisk in the yogurt and mix well. Keep in a covered container in the refrigerator for up to a week. (Makes 1 cup.)

Curried Low-Fat Vinaigrette

Use the recipe above. Omit the herbs. Add ½ teaspoon ground cumin and ½ teaspoon curry powder or more, to taste.

Tomato Vinaigrette

Use the recipe for Yogurt Vinaigrette, but substitute either 1 ripe tomato or ¾ cup tomato juice for the yogurt. Blend all the ingredients together in a blender.

Tofu Vinaigrette

Juice of ½ lemon
  2 tablespoons wine or cider vinegar
½ cup plain low-fat yogurt
  1 small clove garlic
  1 teaspoon Dijon style mustard
  1 teaspoon soy sauce

Protein ++
Potassium +
Minerals +

¼ pound tofu
Freshly ground pepper to taste

Place all the ingredients in a blender or food processor and blend together until completely smooth. (Makes 1 cup.)

Low-Fat Green Goddess Dressing

To either the Tofu Vinaigrette, above, or the Yogurt Vinaigrette, add ½ cup parsley or spinach, washed and dried. Blend together all the ingredients in a food processor or blender until completely smooth. (Makes 1½ cups.)

Marinated Vegetables

Every few days make a bowl of these marinated vegetables to have on hand in the refrigerator for easy, delicious, healthy snacks and sandwiches.

½ pound mushrooms, cut in halves or quarters if large

Potassium + +
Fiber +
Vitamin C +
Minerals +

1 cucumber, peeled and sliced
1 zucchini, sliced
1 cauliflower, broken into florets and steamed 5 minutes
1 bunch broccoli, broken into florets and steamed 5 minutes
1 green pepper, sliced in rings
1 red pepper, sliced in rings
1 red onion, sliced in rings

For the marinade:
½ cup wine or cider vinegar
Juice of 1 lemon
1 clove garlic, minced or put through a press
1 tablespoon Dijon mustard
½ teaspoon tarragon
½ teaspoon thyme or marjoram
2 tablespoons chopped fresh herbs, such as dill, basil, parsley, or oregano
Freshly ground pepper to taste
¼ cup olive oil
1 cup water

Prepare the vegetables and place in a bowl.

Stir together the vinegar, lemon juice, garlic, mustard, and herbs. Add freshly ground pepper to taste. Whisk in the olive oil and the water and combine thoroughly. Pour over the vegetables and toss together. Cover and refrigerate. This will keep for several days. (Serves 6.)

Warm Vegetable Salad

1 Bermuda onion, cut in rings	Complex carbohydrate +++
½ pound new potatoes, diced	Vitamin A +
½ bunch broccoli, cut in florets	Magnesium +
½ head cauliflower, cut in florets	
¼ pound mushrooms, cleaned, trimmed, and quartered	
12 cherry tomatoes	
¼ pound tofu (optional), diced and tossed with soy sauce	
1 recipe Yogurt Vinaigrette (page 219)	
¼ cup chopped fresh parsley or other herbs	
2–3 tablespoons freshly grated Parmesan	

Place the onion and potatoes in a steamer above boiling water and steam 10 minutes. Add the broccoli, cauliflower, and mushrooms and continue to steam for 5 to 10 minutes, depending on how crunchy you want your vegetables. Remove from the heat, refresh under cold water, and toss at once with the remaining ingredients. Serve warm. (Serves 6 to 8.)

Vegetable Salad Sandwiches or Pita Pockets

For sandwiches, use the above recipe (or leftovers from the above recipe). Use ¼ cup per sandwich, or more for pita pockets (up to ½ cup), and top with 1 tablespoon grated swiss or cheddar cheese. For a delicious hot open-faced sandwich, top whole-grain bread with the mixture and 1 tablespoon grated cheese, and run under the broiler until the cheese melts.

Mixed Bean Salad

1½ cups cooked garbanzo beans
    (½ cup raw dried, or
    use canned)
1½ cups cooked kidney beans
    (½ cup dried, or use canned)
1½ cups cooked navy beans or
    black beans (½ cup dried,
    or use canned)
1 large green pepper, chopped
1 small onion, chopped, *or*
4 green onions, chopped
4 to 6 radishes, sliced
3 tablespoons chopped fresh cilantro

Protein +++
Complex carbohydrate +++
Fiber ++

For the dressing:

¼ cup wine or cider vinegar
1 clove garlic, minced or put through a press
1 teaspoon Dijon style mustard
½–1 teaspoon ground cumin, to taste
¾ cup liquid from the beans
Salt and freshly ground pepper to taste

Mix together the beans, green pepper, onion, radishes, and cilantro.

For the dressing, mix together the vinegar, garlic, mustard, and cumin. Stir in the liquid from the beans and combine well. Add salt and freshly ground pepper to taste.

Toss the dressing with the beans and serve, or chill and serve. This makes a good school lunch in a jar. (Serves 6 to 8.)

Warm Garbanzo Bean Salad

2 cups garbanzo beans, washed and
    picked over
6 cups water
    Salt to taste
4 green onions, chopped
4 radishes, chopped
1 green or red pepper, chopped
½ cup chopped fresh parsley
¼ cup freshly grated Parmesan or
    cheddar cheese

Protein +++
Complex carbohydrate ++
Vitamin A ++
Vitamin C +

1 recipe Yogurt Vinaigrette, either plain
  or with cumin or curry to taste (page
  219)
Freshly ground pepper to taste
Leaf lettuce, washed and dried, for
serving

Pick over the beans, wash, and soak for several hours or
overnight in the 6 cups water. Drain and place in a large pot
with another 6 cups water. Bring to a boil, cover, and reduce
heat. Cook 1 to 2 hours, until soft, adding salt to taste halfway
through the cooking.

Drain the beans and toss with the green onions, radishes,
green or red pepper, parsley, and grated cheese. Toss again with
the Yogurt Vinaigrette of your choice and season to taste with
freshly ground pepper. Serve warm, on plates or from a bowl
lined with lettuce leaves. (Serves 6.)

Note: You can use canned garbanzos for this. Simply heat
the beans in their liquid, drain, and toss with the remaining
ingredients.

Broccoli Salad

1 large bunch broccoli (1½–   Complex carbohydrate + +
  2 pounds), broken into florets,   Protein + +
  stems peeled and chopped   Potassium + +
4 green onions, chopped
2 tablespoons freshly grated Parmesan
  or gruyère cheese
2–4 tablespoons chopped fresh parsley or
  other herbs
¼ pound tofu, diced and tossed with
  soy sauce (optional)
Low-Fat Vinaigrette of your choice
(pages 219–220)

Steam the broccoli for 5 to 8 minutes. Refresh under cold
water and shake dry.

Toss with the remaining salad ingredients and the dressing
of your choice. Serve, or chill and serve. (Serves 4.)

Grated Carrot Salad

2 pounds carrots, peeled and grated   Vitamin A + + +
1/4–1/2 cup chopped fresh parsley   Vitamin C + + +
1 recipe Yogurt Vinaigrette or Curried Yogurt
   Vinaigrette (page 219)

Toss together the carrots, parsley, and dressing. Serve right away or refrigerate. This will keep for a couple of days in the refrigerator. (Serves 4 to 6.)

Carrot Apple Salad

For the salad: Complex carbohydrate +
1 pound carrots, scrubbed and grated   Vitamin A + + +
1 pound apples, grated   Vitamin C +
3 tablespoons currants

For the dressing:
Juice of 1/2 lemon
2 tablespoons cider vinegar
1 tablespoon honey
Pinch of salt
1/2 cup plain low-fat yogurt

Toss together the carrots, apples, and currants.
Blend together the lemon juice, vinegar, honey, and salt. Stir in the yogurt. Toss with the carrots, apples, and currants and serve. (Serves 4 to 6.)

Chinese Chicken Salad

2 cups diced cooked chicken breast   Protein + + +
1 green pepper, chopped   Vitamin C +
4 green onions, chopped   Complex carbohydrate +
2 tablespoons sunflower seeds or sesame
   seeds
1/2 cup chopped cucumber
3 tablespoons chopped cilantro

For the dressing:
1/4 cup white wine or cider vinegar, or
   lemon juice
1 tablespoon soy sauce

1 clove garlic, minced or put through a
    press
2 teaspoons freshly grated ginger (or ½
    teaspoon dried)
Freshly ground pepper to taste
2 tablespoons sesame oil
½ cup plain low-fat yogurt

Toss together the chicken, green pepper, green onions, sunflower or sesame seeds, cucumber, and cilantro.

Mix together the vinegar or lemon juice, the soy sauce, garlic, and ginger. Add freshly ground pepper to taste. Whisk in the sesame oil and the yogurt. Toss with the salad and serve, or refrigerate and serve. This makes a good school lunch in a jar and will last a day or two in the refrigerator. (Serves 4.)

Low-Fat Egg Salad

4 hard-boiled eggs, chopped   Protein +++
Whites only of 4 additional hard-boiled eggs,   Vitamin C +
    chopped
1 green pepper, minced
1 small onion, minced
1 stalk celery, minced
3 tablespoons chopped fresh parsley (optional)
1 recipe Tofu Vinaigrette (page 219)
1-3 Additional teaspoons mustard
Freshly ground pepper to taste
½ teaspoon paprika or curry powder (optional)

Toss together the chopped eggs and egg whites with the vegetables, parsley, Tofu Vinaigrette, additional mustard, ground pepper, and optional paprika or curry powder. Store in the refrigerator in a covered container, and use for sandwiches or salads. (Serves 4.)

Escarole and Orange Salad

½ pound escarole lettuce, leaves   Vitamin C ++
    separated, washed well and dried   Complex carbohydrate ++
3 green onions, sliced
4 radishes, cleaned and thinly sliced
4 mushrooms, cleaned, trimmed, and sliced

    2 oranges, peel and white pith removed,
      cut in sections
    2 tablespoons sunflower or sesame seeds
    1 recipe Yogurt Vinaigrette (page 219)

Toss together the escarole, green onions, mushrooms, radishes, sunflower or sesame seeds, and oranges with the dressing and serve. (Serves 4 to 6.)

Note: You may add juice of ½ orange to the dressing for more orange flavor.

Cottage Fruit Salad

2 cups low-fat cottage cheese	Calcium +++
1 apple, chopped	Protein +++
1 banana or pear, chopped	Vitamin C ++
½ cup chopped fresh pineapple	
3 tablespoons sunflower seeds	
2 tablespoons raisins	

Toss all the ingredients together and chill until ready to serve. (Serves 4.)

Lentil Salad

1 cup lentils, washed and picked over	Protein +++
1 small onion, chopped	Complex carbohydrate ++
2 cloves garlic, minced	
1 bay leaf	
3 cups water	

Salt to taste
¾ cup Yogurt Vinaigrette (page 219)
½ teaspoon ground cumin (optional)
    1 small green pepper, chopped
    3 green onions, chopped
Freshly ground pepper to taste
Optional: chopped fresh herbs, such
         as parsley, thyme, basil,
         coriander

Combine the lentils, onion, garlic, bay leaf, and water and bring to a boil. Cover, reduce heat, and simmer 45 minutes, until tender. Add salt to taste. Drain off excess liquid (save for soups) and remove the bay leaf.

Mix together the ingredients for the dressing and stir in the optional cumin. Toss with the lentils, green pepper, green onions, and optional herbs. Add plenty of freshly ground pepper. Serve warm, or chill several hours in a covered container. This makes a good lunch in a jar and will keep for 5 days in the refrigerator. (Serves 4.)

Mexican Salad

2 cups cooked corn kernels (from 4 ears of corn, or may use frozen)
1 green pepper, chopped
1 jalapeño pepper, chopped
1 small onion, chopped
½ red pepper, chopped
3 tablespoons chopped cilantro
⅓ cup cubed or grated skim milk mozzarella or farmer cheese
1 recipe Yogurt Vinaigrette with ½ 1 teaspoon ground cumin (page 219)

Complex carbohydrate +++
Calcium ++
Vitamin C +

Toss together all the vegetables, the cilantro, and the cheese with the dressing and serve, or chill and serve. This would make a good school lunch in a jar. (Serves 4.)

Middle Eastern Salad

1 small cucumber, peeled and chopped
1 green pepper, chopped
4 tomatoes, chopped
4 green onions, chopped
1 tablespoon chopped fresh dill, if available

Vitamin A +++
Vitamin C +++

For the dressing:
Juice of 1 large lemon
1 small clove garlic, minced or put through a press
1 teaspoon Dijon mustard (optional)
½ cup plain low-fat yogurt
Freshly ground pepper to taste

Toss together the vegetables and dill.

Mix together the lemon juice, garlic, and mustard. Stir in the yogurt and combine well. Add freshly ground pepper to taste. Serve at once, or chill and serve. (Serves 4 to 6.)

Bulgur Pilaf Salad

¼–½ pound tofu, to taste
Soy sauce
   2 cups Bulgar Pilaf (page 260)
   2 cups steamed broccoli, chopped
   2 tomatoes, chopped
Juice of 2 lemons
   1 clove garlic, minced or put through a press
   1 teaspoon mustard
   ½ cup plain low-fat yogurt
Freshly ground pepper to taste

Protein +++
Complex carbohydrate ++
Vitamin A ++
Calcium +

Mash the tofu with the soy sauce and toss with the bulgur, broccoli, and tomatoes.

Mix together the lemon juice, garlic, mustard, yogurt, and freshly ground pepper and toss with the bulgur mixture. Refrigerate until ready to eat. This will keep for a couple of days in the refrigerator. (Serves 4 to 6.)

Warm Potato Salad

1½ pounds new or russet potatoes
   ¼ cup dry white wine
   1 Bermuda onion, thinly sliced
   1 green pepper, chopped
   2 teaspoons caraway seeds (optional)
   ¼ cup chopped fresh parsley
   3 tablespoons freshly grated Parmesan (optional)
Freshly ground pepper to taste
   1 recipe Yogurt Vinaigrette (page 219)

Complex carbohydrate +++
Vitamin C ++
Vitamin A ++

Cut the potatoes in half if large and steam until just tender, about 20 minutes. Refresh under cold water, dice and toss with the white wine. Add the Bermuda onion, green pepper, optional caraway seeds, parsley, and optional Parmesan. Add freshly ground pepper to taste.

Mix together the Yogurt Vinaigrette, toss with the salad, and serve.

Note: You can vary the flavor of this salad by adding 1 teaspoon curry powder or 1 teaspoon ground cumin to the vinaigrette. (Serves 6.)

Curried Brown Rice Salad

1 cup raw brown rice, cooked	Complex carbohydrate +++
3 green onions, chopped	Vitamin C +
1 stalk celery, chopped	Vitamin A +
½ cup chopped cucumber	Calcium +
1 small bell pepper, chopped	
3 tablespoons grated Parmesan cheese	
2 tablespoons sunflower seeds	
¾–1 cup Curried Low-Fat Vinaigrette (page 219)	

Cook the brown rice and toss with the remaining ingredients. Refrigerate for at least one hour in a covered container. This makes a good lunch in a jar and will keep for 3 days in the refrigerator.

Spinach Salad

½ pound fresh spinach, washed carefully, stems removed, and dried	Complex carbohydrate ++
4–6 mushrooms, cleaned, stems trimmed, and sliced	Potassium ++
2 green onions (optional), sliced	Protein ++
2 tomatoes (optional), cut in wedges	
1 cup alfalfa sprouts	
¼ cup roasted soybeans (below)	
Low-Fat Vinaigrette of your choice (pages 219–220)	

Combine all the ingredients for the salad and toss with the dressing of your choice just before serving. (Serves 4 to 6.)

To roast soybeans: Soak 1 cup overnight in 3 cups water. Drain and cook 1 hour in 3 cups water. Drain. Bake 1 hour at 325° or until toasty and cooked through.

Spinach and Tangerine Salad

½ pound spinach, washed,
  stems removed, dried
4 mushrooms, cleaned, trimmed,
  and sliced
2–3 tangerines, peeled, sectioned
1 cup alfalfa sprouts
1 recipe Yogurt Vinaigrette (page 219)

Complex carbohydrate ++
Vitamin A ++
Vitamin C ++

Toss together the spinach, mushrooms, tangerines, and alfalfa sprouts with the dressing and serve. (Serves 4 to 6.)

Oriental Sprouts Salad

For the salad:
1 cup alfalfa sprouts
2 cups mung bean sprouts
2 tablespoons sunflower seeds
2 carrots, grated
2–3 green onions, minced
2 tablespoons chopped cilantro

Complex carbohydrate +++
Vitamin A ++
Protein +

For the dressing:
1 tablespoon sesame tahini
1 tablespoon soy sauce
4 tablespoons cider vinegar
1 teaspoon grated fresh ginger
1 clove garlic, minced or put through
  a press
1 teaspoon Dijon mustard
Freshly ground pepper to taste
2 tablespoons sesame or safflower oil
¾ cup plain low-fat yogurt or vegetable
  stock (page 242)

Toss together the ingredients for the salad.

Mix together the sesame tahini, soy sauce, vinegar, ginger, garlic, mustard, and pepper. Whisk in the oil and the yogurt or vegetable stock. Blend well and toss with the sprouts. Serve at once or chill in a covered container. (Serves 4 to 6.)

Tofu Sprouts Salad

    4 ounces tofu
Soy sauce to taste
    2 cups bean sprouts
    1 small green pepper, chopped
    3 green onions, chopped
    1 tomato, chopped
    1 tablespoon sesame or sunflower seeds
      (optional)
2–3 tablespoons chopped fresh cilantro or
      other fresh herbs (optional)
½–1 teaspoon grated fresh ginger (optional)
    ¾ cup Yogurt Vinaigrette, Curried Yogurt
      Vinaigrette, or Tofu Vinaigrette (page
      219)

Protein +++
Vitamin C +
Complex carbohydrate +

Place the tofu in a bowl and mash with the soy sauce. Toss with the remaining ingredients. Refrigerate in a covered bowl. Use for sandwiches, on whole grain bread or pita bread, or as a salad. (Serves 4.)

Tabouli

1½ cups bulgur wheat
Boiling water to cover
    1 small cucumber, chopped
    4 green onions, chopped
    1 cup chopped fresh parsley
    3 tablespoons chopped fresh mint
    4 tomatoes, chopped
Juice to 2 large lemons (more to
    taste)
    1 clove garlic, minced or put through
    a press
    1 teaspoon Dijon mustard
    ½ teaspoon ground cumin (optional)
Salt and freshly ground pepper to
    taste
    2 tablespoons olive oil
    ½ cup plain low-fat yogurt

Complex carbohydrate +++
Protein ++
Vitamin A ++
Vitamin C ++

Place the bulgur in a bowl and pour on boiling water to cover by about 1 inch. Prepare the vegetables and dressing while the bulgur "cooks" in the water.

For the dressing, mix together the lemon juice, garlic, Dijon mustard, the optional cumin, and the salt and freshly ground pepper. Whisk in the olive oil and the yogurt.

When the bulgur is soft, pour off any excess water and press the bulgur in a strainer or squeeze in a towel. Then toss with the cucumber, onions, parsley, mint, tomatoes, and the dressing. Taste and adjust seasonings, adding more lemon juice, garlic, mustard, or salt and pepper if you wish. Refrigerate several hours, or serve at once.

This will keep several days in the refrigerator and makes a good school lunch in a jar. (Serves 6.)

Tomato Salad

4 large, firm, ripe tomatoes, sliced thin	Vitamin C +++ Complex carbohydrate ++
2 tablespoons chopped fresh herbs, such as basil, parsley, thyme, marjoram, or dill	
2 tablespoons red wine vinegar	
1 small clove garlic, minced or put through a press	
½–1 teaspoon Dijon mustard, to taste	
1 tablespoon olive oil	
2 tablespoons safflower oil (can use all safflower oil)	
Freshly ground pepper to taste	

Slice the tomatoes and line a serving platter with them. Sprinkle with the herbs.

Mix together the vinegar, garlic, and mustard, and whisk in the oils. Drizzle this over the tomatoes and add freshly ground pepper to taste. Serve at once, or chill and serve. (Serves 4 to 6.)

Watercress and Mushroom Salad

2 bunches (about 4 cups) watercress, washed, dried, stems trimmed	Vitamin A +++ Vitamin C + Complex carbohydrate ++
¼ pound mushrooms, trimmed, cleaned, and sliced thin	

        2 tablespoons shelled walnuts or pecans
        1 recipe Yogurt Vinaigrette (page 219) or
            Tofu Vinaigrette (page 219)
    ½ cup alfalfa sprouts

Toss together the watercress, mushrooms, and walnuts or pecans with the dressing just before serving. Garnish with the alfalfa sprouts. (Serves 4 to 6.)

Soups

White Bean Soup with Whole-Grain Croutons

2 cups white beans, washed, picked over, and soaked overnight	Protein +++ Complex carbohydrate +++

        1 onion, chopped
        3 cloves garlic, minced or put through a press
        1 tablespoon safflower oil
        6 cups water
        1 bay leaf
    ½ teaspoon thyme
1–2 teaspoons salt, to taste
Freshly ground pepper to taste
Up to 1 cup skim milk (optional)
Juice of 1 large lemon
    ¼ cup chopped fresh parsley
    1½ cups whole-grain croutons
        (instructions below)

Heat the oil in a large, heavy-bottomed soup pot or Dutch oven and sauté the onion and 2 cloves of the garlic until the onion is tender.

Drain the soaked beans and add to the pot, along with the water and bay leaf. Bring to a boil, reduce heat, and simmer 1½ hours. Add the thyme, salt and pepper to taste, and the remaining garlic, and continue to simmer another 30 minutes to an hour, until the beans are thoroughly tender. Remove the bay leaf and puree the soup in a blender. Return to the pot and heat through. Add freshly ground pepper to taste and adjust salt. If you wish, thin out to desired consistency with skim milk.

* Make the croutons while the soup is simmering. Cut whole-grain bread into small squares and bake in 325° oven until brown and crisp. Remove from the heat.

Just before serving the soup, stir in the lemon juice. Serve, topping each bowl with parsley and whole-grain croutons. (Serves 6.)

White Bean Soup Using Canned Beans

Follow the recipe above. Substitute for the beans and water:

4 cups canned white beans
2 cups water

Proceed as in the recipe above, sautéing the onion and garlic in the oil, and adding the beans and their liquid. But you needn't bring this to a simmer. Puree and return to the pot. Proceed as above.

Cabbage Soup à la Chinoise

5 cups vegetable stock or bouillon (page 242)	Protein + + Complex carbohydrate + +
4 cups shredded Chinese cabbage	
6 green onions, thinly sliced	
¼ cup soy sauce	
2 tablespoons sherry	
1 teaspoon grated fresh ginger	
½–1 pound tofu, cut in cubes or slivers (optional)	
2 tablespoons sesame seeds, for garnish	

Place the stock in a large soup pot and bring to a simmer. Add the Chinese cabbage and green onions and simmer 5 minutes, until the cabbage is cooked through but still has some texture. Stir in the remaining ingredients, heat through and serve. (Serves 4 to 6.)

Cabbage Apple Soup

1 tablespoon safflower oil	Complex carbohydrate + + +
1 large onion, chopped	Calcium + +
2 cloves garlic, minced or put through a press	Vitamin A +

    4 cups shredded red or green cabbage
    6 cups water or vegetable stock (page 242)
1–2 teaspoons curry powder
    2 tablespoons soy sauce
Salt to taste
    2 tart apples, cored and sliced
    1 cup plain low-fat yogurt
Freshly ground pepper to taste

For garnish:
½ cup additional yogurt
½ additional apple, sliced thin and tossed
    with lemon juice

Heat the safflower oil in a heavy-bottomed soup pot or Dutch oven and sauté the onion and garlic over medium heat until the onion begins to soften. Add the cabbage and sauté another 5 minutes, stirring. Add the water or stock, the curry powder, soy sauce, and salt to taste. Bring to a boil, reduce heat, cover, and simmer 30 minutes. Add the apples and continue to simmer another 15 to 20 minutes. Taste and adjust seasoning, adding more salt or curry powder to taste. Remove from the heat, cool a minute, and stir in the yogurt and freshly ground pepper to taste. Serve, topping each bowlful with a spoonful of yogurt and a few slices of apple. (Serves 4 to 6.)

Curried Cauliflower Soup

    1 onion, chopped
    1 clove garlic, minced or put
      through a press
    1 tablespoon safflower oil
1–2 teaspoons curry powder, to taste
½–1 teaspoon ground cumin, to taste
    1 small head (about 4 cups)
      cauliflower, broken into
      florets
    5 cups vegetable or chicken stock or
      bouillon (page 242)
    1 small potato, peeled and diced
Salt and pepper to taste
    1 cup plain low-fat yogurt
    1 teaspoon cornstarch
Lemon juice to taste (optional)

Complex carbohydrate ++
Calcium ++
Magnesium +
Protein +

Heat the oil in a soup pot and sauté the onion and garlic until the onion is tender. Add the curry powder, cumin, and cauliflower, stir together for a minute or two, and add the stock or bouillon and the potato and bring to a boil. Cover, reduce heat, and simmer 30 minutes. Puree in a blender or food processor, in batches. Return to the pot and adjust seasonings, adding salt, pepper, and curry powder or cumin to taste. Heat through.

Stir together the yogurt and cornstarch and whisk into the soup. If you like, whisk in the optional lemon juice. Heat through and serve. (Serves 4 to 6.)

Chicken Noodle or Tofu Noodle Soup

6 cups vegetable stock or chicken stock   Protein +++
         Complex carbohydrate ++
8 ounces diced or shredded chicken or tofu
8 ounces flat whole wheat noodles or spaghetti
2 eggs, beaten
Juice of 1½ lemons
3 green onions, green part only, thinly sliced
Freshly ground pepper to taste

Simmer the vegetable or chicken stock and add the chicken or tofu. Simmer for about 10 to 15 minutes, until cooked through, and add the noodles or spaghetti. Simmer until the pasta is cooked al dente, still firm to the bite.

Beat the eggs in a bowl and add the lemon juice. Stir together, then ladle in some of the simmering stock. Stir this back into the soup, being careful not to boil. Add freshly ground pepper to taste, and serve, topping each bowl with the sliced green onions. (Serves 4 to 6.)

Corn Chowder

1 tablespoon safflower oil   Complex carbohydrate ++
1 onion, chopped   Potassium ++
1 medium or large green pepper, chopped   Calcium ++
         Fiber +
2 medium-sized potatoes, scrubbed and diced

    3 cups fresh or frozen corn kernels (from
        4 or 5 ears corn)
    4 cups water or vegetable stock (page 242)
    ½ teaspoon thyme
    3 cups skim milk
    ½ cup grated Swiss cheese
    Salt and freshly ground pepper to taste

For garnish: ¼ cup chopped fresh parsley or cilantro

Heat the oil in a heavy-bottomed soup pot or Dutch oven and sauté the onion and green pepper until the onion is tender. Add the potatoes, corn, and water or vegetable stock, and bring to a boil. Reduce heat, cover, and simmer 45 minutes. Puree the soup in a blender or food processor. Return to the pot and add the thyme, milk, and salt and freshly ground pepper to taste. Heat through for about 10 minutes, and stir in the grated cheese. Correct seasonings and serve, topping each bowl with chopped fresh parsley or coriander (cilantro). (Serves 6 to 8.)

Blender Gazpacho

This is great to have on hand in the refrigerator, not just for quick lunches but for snacks as well. Make a big bowl of it at the beginning of the week, and you'll be drinking salads all week long. It keeps well and is always refreshing.

    1½ pounds ripe tomatoes, peeled   Complex carbohydrate +++
    1–2 cloves garlic, to taste   Vitamin A +++
    ½ onion   Vitamin C ++
    1 carrot, coarsely chopped
    1 small cucumber, peeled and
        coarsely chopped
    1 green pepper, seeded and coarsely
        chopped
    2 sprigs fresh parsley
    3–4 tablespoons fresh basil, if available
    Juice of 1–2 lemons, to taste
    Salt and freshly ground pepper to taste
    3–4 cups V-8 or tomato juice,
        depending on how thick you want it

Optional: ¼ pound tofu, diced
A handful of alfalfa sprouts
2 tablespoons sunflower seeds
1 cup plain low-fat yogurt

Blend together all except the optional ingredients in a blender until smooth. Chill several hours. Adjust seasonings.

Serve, using the optional ingredients as garnishes. If you are taking this to school in a jar, just add the optional ingredients to each serving and mix together before putting in the jar. (Serves 6 to 8.)

Hearty Lentil Soup

1 tablespoon safflower oil	Complex carbohydrates ++
1 onion, chopped	Protein ++
3 cloves garlic, minced or put	Potassium ++
through a press	Fiber +
2 cups lentils, washed and picked over	
2 carrots, chopped	
2 potatoes, chopped	
2 tomatoes, chopped	
6 cups water	
1 bay leaf	
1 teaspoon cumin	
½ teaspoon oregano or thyme	
Salt and freshly ground pepper to taste	
More water as needed	
Chopped fresh parsley for garnish	

Heat the oil in a heavy bottomed soup pot and add the onion and 2 cloves of the garlic. Sauté until the onion is tender and add the lentils, carrots, potatoes, tomatoes, water, bay leaf, and cumin. Bring to a boil, reduce heat, cover, and simmer 30 minutes. Add the remaining garlic, salt to taste, and lots of freshly ground pepper, and simmer another 15 to 30 minutes. Add more water if necessary. Remove 2 cups of the soup and puree in a blender. Stir back into the soup. Heat through, correct seasonings, and serve, garnishing each serving with chopped fresh parsley. (Serves 4 to 6.)

Minestrone

This can be a week-long soup. Every day add more vegetables and water, and you can keep it going.

1 tablespoon safflower oil	Vitamin A ++
1 onion, chopped	Vitamin C +
3–4 cloves garlic, minced or put through	Calcium ++
a press	Magnesium ++

1 tablespoon safflower oil
1 onion, chopped
3–4 cloves garlic, minced or put through
   a press
2 carrots, sliced
½ small green cabbage, shredded
2 potatoes, scrubbed and diced
1 pound canned or fresh tomatoes, sliced
4 tablespoons tomato paste
2 quarts vegetable stock (page 241) or water
1 rind from Parmesan cheese, if available (optional)
1 bay leaf
1 teaspoon oregano
½ teaspoon thyme
Salt and freshly ground pepper to taste
1 teaspoon dried basil (or 1 tablespoon fresh)
2 cups cooked navy beans or garbanzos
2 zucchini, sliced
1 cup fresh or frozen peas
¼ pound broken spaghetti or flat noodles
1 cup freshly grated Parmesan (or Swiss) cheese
¼ cup chopped fresh parsley

Heat the oil in a large, heavy-bottomed soup pot or Dutch oven and add the onion and garlic. Sauté until the onion is tender, then add the carrots and cabbage. Sauté for about one minute and add the potatoes, tomatoes, tomato paste, and vegetable stock or water. Bring to a simmer and add the optional rind of Parmesan (this gives the soup a great cheesy flavor without additional cheese), the bay leaf, oregano, thyme, salt, basil, and cooked beans. Simmer, covered, for one hour. Taste and adjust seasonings, adding more garlic, salt, or herbs if you wish. Season with lots of freshly ground pepper.

Add the zucchini and peas and simmer 10 to 15 minutes. Add the spaghetti and continue to simmer until the pasta is cooked al dente, firm to the bite. Serve, topping each bowl with

Parmesan or Swiss cheese and chopped fresh parsley. (Serves 6 to 8.)

Split Pea Soup

2 cups split peas, washed and picked over	Protein ++ Complex carbohydrate ++
1 tablespoon safflower oil	
1 onion, chopped	
2 cloves garlic, minced or put through a press	
2 stalks celery, chopped	
1 carrot, chopped	
8 cups water	
1 bay leaf	
½ teaspoon thyme	
Salt and freshly ground pepper to taste	
½ cup plain low-fat yogurt	

Heat the safflower oil in a heavy-bottomed soup pot or Dutch oven and sauté the onion and one clove of the garlic until the onion is tender. Add the carrot and celery, sauté for another minute, and add the split peas, water, and bay leaf. Bring to a boil, reduce heat, and simmer one hour. Add the remaining garlic, the thyme, and salt to taste, and simmer another 30 minutes. Puree half the soup in a blender and return to the pot. Heat through, adjust seasonings, adding salt or garlic if you wish and lots of freshly ground pepper. Serve piping hot, topping each bowl with a spoonful of yogurt. (Serves 6.)

Potato Leek Soup

1 tablespoon safflower oil	Complex carbohydrate ++
4 leeks, white part only, washed well and sliced	Calcium ++ Magnesium ++
2 quarts vegetable stock (page 242) or bouillon	
2 pounds potatoes, scrubbed and diced	
¼ teaspoon thyme	
Salt and freshly ground pepper to taste	
3 tablespoons dry white wine	
¼ cup grated Swis or Parmesan cheese	
Fresh chopped parsley for garnish	

Heat the oil in a heavy-bottomed soup pot and sauté the leeks over low heat, stirring from time to time, for 10 to 15 minutes. Add the vegetable stock, potatoes, and thyme, and bring to a simmer. Cover and simmer 30 minutes. Add salt and freshly ground pepper to taste, and the wine. Correct seasonings and serve, topping each bowlful with grated cheese and chopped fresh parsley. (Serves 4 to 6.)

Puree of Spinach Soup

1 tablespoon safflower oil
1 small onion, chopped
1 clove garlic, minced or put through a press
1 pound fresh spinach, washed, stemmed, and chopped, *or*
1 10-ounce package frozen spinach
1 large potato, peeled and diced
3 cups water or vegetable stock (see below)
Salt and freshly ground pepper to taste
2 cups skim milk
¼ teaspoon nutmeg
½ cup freshly grated Parmesan or Swisscheese
½ cup plain low-fat yogurt

Complex carbohydrate + +
Calcium + +
Potassium + +

Heat the safflower oil in a large, heavy-bottomed soup pot or Dutch oven and sauté the onion and garlic until the onion is tender. Add the spinach, potato, and water or stock and bring to a boil. Add salt to taste, reduce heat, cover, and simmer for 20 minutes, or until the potato is tender. Puree in a blender or put through a food mill and return to the pot. Add the milk and nutmeg and heat through. Add freshly ground pepper to taste, stir in the cheese, and serve, topping each bowl with a dollop of low-fat yogurt. (Serves 4.)

Vegetable Stock

This recipe is taken from *Herb and Honey Cookery*, by Martha Rose Shulman.

2 quarts water   Vitamin A + +
2 onions, quartered   Calcium +
6 cloves garlic, peeled   Magnesium +
2 carrots, coarsely sliced
2 leeks, white part only, cleaned and coarsely sliced
2 potatoes, scrubbed and quartered
2 stalks celery, coarsely sliced
2 sprigs parsley
1 bay leaf
¼ teaspoon thyme
Salt to taste
12 black peppercorns

Combine all the ingredients in a soup pot and bring to a simmer. Cover, reduce heat, and simmer 1 to 2 hours. Strain and discard the vegetables. This can be frozen and will last for several days in the refrigerator. (Makes 2 quarts.)

Easy Vegetable Bouillon

2 quarts water
4 vegetable bouillon cubes (available in natural foods stores and some supermarkets)
4 tablespoons soy sauce (more to taste)

Simmer the above ingredients together until the bouillon cubes dissolve. (Makes 2 quarts.)

For Dinner: Main Dishes and Side Dishes

Chicken and Fish

Ronnie's Broiled Chicken Breasts

4 3–4-ounce chicken breasts, skins removed   Protein + + +
1 teaspoon safflower or olive oil
Juice of 1 lemon
1 large clove garlic, minced or put through a press
½ teaspoon thyme
½ teaspoon paprika
Freshly ground pepper to taste
½ teaspoon cumin (optional)

Preheat the broiler.

Brush the chicken breasts with olive or safflower oil, sprinkle with the lemon juice, and top with the garlic and herbs. Add freshly ground pepper to taste.

Broil for 5 to 7 minutes on each side, until cooked through, and serve. (Serves 4.)

Chicken and Vegetable Curry

1 tablespoon safflower oil
8–10 ounces chicken breast, diced
1 onion, sliced
1 clove garlic, minced or put
  through a press
1 tablespoon grated fresh ginger
1–2 teaspoons curry powder, or more, to
  taste
½–1 teaspoon ground cumin, to taste
1 large carrot, sliced
1–2 cups shredded red cabbage
1 zucchini, sliced
Water
Salt and freshly ground pepper to taste
1 cup plain low-fat yogurt
1 teaspoon cornstarch

Protein +++
Complex carbohydrate +
Vitamin A +
Calcium +

Heat the oil in a nonstick skillet and sauté the diced chicken breast until cooked through. Remove from heat and add the onion, garlic, ginger, cumin, and curry powder. Sauté until the onion is tender, and add the carrot and a couple tablespoons of water. Cook, stirring, another 5 minutes, adding a little water if necessary, and add the cabbage and zucchini. Continue to cook for another 5 to 10 minutes, until the zucchini is bright green and cooked through, Stir the chicken back into the pan and add a little salt and pepper.

Mix together the yogurt and cornstarch and stir into the vegetable and chicken mixture. Taste and adjust seasonings, adding more curry powder, cumin, or salt if you wish. Heat

through and serve over hot cooked grains, such as bulgur or
brown rice. (Serves 4.)

Stir-Fried Chicken and Vegetables

1 tablespoon safflower oil	Protein +++
8–10 ounces chicken breast, diced	Complex carbohydrate ++
1 onion, sliced	Vitamin A ++
1 clove garlic, minced or put through a press	
1 tablespoon grated fresh ginger	
1 large carrot, sliced	
1–2 cups regular or Chinese cabbage, shredded	
2 tablespoons sesame or sunflower seeds	
1 zucchini, sliced, or broccoli florets	
1 tomato, chopped	
½ teaspoon basil	
2 tablespoons soy sauce	
1 teaspoon vinegar	
1 teaspoon honey	
¼ cup water	
1 tablespoon cornstarch	

Heat the oil in a nonstick skillet and sauté the diced chicken
breast over medium-high heat until cooked through. Remove
from heat and add the onion, garlic, and ginger. Sauté until the
onion is tender, and add the carrot and a couple of tablespoons
of water. Cook, stirring, for about 5 minutes, and add the cabbage and sesame or sunflower seeds. Cook, stirring another 5
minutes, adding a little water if necessary. Add the zucchini or
broccoli and sauté another 5 minutes, then stir in the tomato,
basil and the cooked chicken. Cover and simmer over medium
heat for 5 minutes. Meanwhile, mix together the soy sauce,
vinegar, honey, water, and cornstarch in a small bowl. Stir into
the chicken-vegetable mixture and continue to cook, stirring,
until the chicken and vegetables are glazed. Remove from the
heat and serve with hot cooked grains, such as brown rice,
bulgur, millet, or couscous. (Serves 4.)

Fish Dishes

Fish Teriyaki

1 pound fish filets (such as flounder, sole, cod,   Protein +++
   or whiting)
2 tablespoons soy sauce
1 tablespoon sherry
1 to 2 teaspoons freshly grated ginger
Juice of ½ lemon
1 tablespoon sesame oil.

Mix together the soy sauce, sherry, ginger, lemon juice, and sesame oil and place in a shallow baking dish. Lay the filets in the dish, cover, and refrigerate for at least 1 hour (and up to a day), turning once or twice.

Preheat the oven to 425°. Bake the fish 8 to 12 minutes, until it is opaque and flakes easily with a fork. Serve hot. (Serves 4.)

Broiled Salmon Steaks

1 tablespoon safflower or sesame oil   Protein +++
2 tablespoons soy sauce   Calcium +
1 teaspoon freshly grated ginger (optional)
1 teaspoon honey (optional)
4 salmon steaks, about ¾ inch thick

Combine the sesame or safflower oil, the soy sauce, ginger, and honey. Marinate the salmon steaks in this mixture while you preheat the broiler for 15 minutes.

Place the salmon 4 inches from the heat. Broil for 4 to 5 minutes on each side, basting once on each side. Serve at once, with wedges of lemon. (Serves 4.)

Sweet and Sour Shrimp

For the sauce: Protein +++
  3 tablespoons cider or white wine   Complex carbohydrate ++
    vinegar
  2 tablespoons honey
  2 tablespoons soy sauce
  ¼ cup water
  1 tablespoon cornstarch or arrowroot

For the shrimp:
    1 pound shrimp, shelled and cleaned
    1 tablespoon safflower oil
    4 green onions, sliced
    1 teaspoon grated fresh ginger (or ¼
        teaspoon powdered)
    1 clove garlic, minced or put through a
        press
    1½ cups frozen peas, thawed (or fresh peas,
        steamed 5–10 minutes, until tender and
        bright green)

First mix together the ingredients for the sauce. Combine the vinegar, honey, soy sauce, and water in a small bowl or measuring cup and stir in the cornstarch or arrowroot. Set aside.

Heat the oil over medium-high heat in a wok or large skillet, preferably nonstick. Add the green onions, ginger, and garlic, and stir-fry 1 minute. Add the shrimp and stir-fry 2 minutes, until pink and cooked through. Add the peas, toss together, and stir in the sauce. Turn down the heat a little and cook, stirring until the shrimp and vegetables are glazed. Serve immediately over hot cooked grains. (Serves 4 to 6.)

Poached Filets of Sole with Tomato Puree

    1 pound filets of sole   Protein +++
    ½ cup dry white wine
    ½ cup water
Juice of 1 lemon

For the tomato puree:
    2 teaspoons safflower oil
    1–2 cloves garlic, minced or put through a press
    2 pounds tomatoes, canned or fresh, seeded and
        chopped
    ½–1 teaspoon dried thyme, oregano, or basil (or 1
        tablespoon chopped fresh basil)
Salt and freshly ground pepper to taste

First make the tomato puree. Heat the safflower oil in a heavy-bottomed frying pan and sauté the garlic over medium-low heat for 1 to 2 minutes, until golden. Add the tomatoes and bring to a simmer. Simmer over medium-low heat, uncovered, for 30 minutes, stirring often. Season to taste with thyme, oregano, or basil, and salt and freshly ground pepper. Mash the sauce with the back of a spoon and set aside.

Now poach the fish. In a wide skillet, saucepan, or casserole that will accommodate all the filets, combine the wine, water, and lemon juice and bring to a simmer. Pound the filets with the flat side of a knife so that they don't curl, and score a couple of times on each side. Gently lower into the simmering broth. Make sure they are submerged, and poach for 10 minutes, or until opaque and the fish flakes easily with a fork. Remove from the liquid with a slotted spoon or spatula and place on a platter or individual plates. Top with the tomato puree, or place the puree on the side, and serve at once. (Serves 4.)

Pasta and Other Meatless Main Dishes

Spaghetti with Tomato Sauce and Parmesan

1 tablespoon safflower or vegetable oil	Complex carbohydrate + +
1 small onion, chopped	Potassium +
2 cloves garlic (more to taste), minced or put through a press	Calcium +
3 pounds ripe tomatoes (fresh or canned) seeded and chopped	
2 tablespoons tomato paste	
Salt to taste	
1 tablespoon fresh chooped basil (or 1 teaspoon dried)	
1 teaspoon oregano	
Freshly ground pepper to taste	
¾ pound whole wheat spaghetti	
2 ounces freshly grated Parmesan cheese	

Heat the safflower or vegetable oil in a heavy-bottomed saucepan or wide skillet and add the onion and garlic. Saute over medium heat until the onion is tender, and add the tomatoes and tomato paste. Bring to a simmer, add salt to taste, cover, and simmer for 30 minutes. Add the herbs and more salt or garlic if you wish, and continue to simmer another 15 minutes.

Meanwhile, bring a large pot of water to a rolling boil. Add some salt and a teaspoon of oil, then add the spaghetti. Cook just until al dente, barely tender to the bite. This will take anywhere from 5 to 10 minutes, depending on the kind of spaghetti you have.

When the spaghetti is cooked, drain and toss immediately with the tomato sauce, or distribute among the plates and spoon sauce over each serving. Serve at once, passing the Parmesan, to be sprinkled over each serving. (Serves 4 to 6.)

Spaghetti with Tofu Tomato Sauce

This spaghetti sauce proves that you don't have to have hamburger to make a hearty, meaty-tasting, high-protein sauce for pasta. Those who are convinced they will never eat tofu won't even recognize this miracle food.

1 tablespoon safflower oil	Protein ++
1 onion, chopped	Complex carbohydrate ++ +
2–4 cloves garlic, to taste, minced	Vitamin A ++
or put through a press	Calcium ++

1 tablespoon safflower oil
1 onion, chopped
2–4 cloves garlic, to taste, minced
   or put through a press
½ pound tofu
1–2 tablespoons soy sauce, to taste
3 pounds fresh (or 2 large cans)
   tomatoes, chopped
1 small can tomato paste
Salt to taste
1–2 teaspoons oregano
½ teaspoon thyme
1–2 tablespoons chooped fresh basil (or
   1 teaspoon dried)
Pinch of cinnamon
Freshly ground pepper to taste
¾ pound whole wheat spaghetti
¼–½ cup freshly grated Parmesan cheese

Heat the safflower oil in a heavy-bottomed casserole or wide frying pan and sauté the onion with half the garlic until the onion is tender. Add the tofu and sauté, mashing with the back of your spoon, for about 5 minutes. Add the soy sauce and continue to sauté another few minutes. Add the tomatoes and bring to a simmer. Add the tomato paste and salt and continue to simmer over low heat, covered, for 30 minutes. Stir in the remaining garlic, the oregano, thyme, basil, and cinnamon, and continue to simmer for 15 to 30 minutes. Adjust seasonings, adding salt, garlic, or herbs if you wish, and plenty of fresh ground pepper.

Bring a large pot of water to a rolling boil, add some salt and the pasta. Cook al dente, until cooked through but still firm to the bite (5–10 minutes, depending on the pasta), drain, and toss immediately with the sauce. Or distribute the pasta among warm plates and spoon the sauce onto each serving. Pass the Parmesan in a bowl and sprinkle on to taste. (Serves 4 to 6.)

Pasta with Cottage Cheese Sauce

2 teaspoons safflower oil
1 onion, chopped
2–3 cloves garlic, minced or put through a press
2 large cans tomatoes, drained and chopped (or 2 pounds fresh tomatoes, chopped)
3 tablespoons tomato paste
1 teaspoon oregano
1 teaspoon basil
Pinch of cinnamon
Salt and freshly ground pepper to taste
2 cups low-fat cottage cheese
¾ pound whole wheat spaghetti or other pasta
½ cup freshly grated Parmesan

Complex carbohydrate ++
Calcium ++
Protein +
Fiber +

Heat the safflower oil in a heavy-bottomed casserole or wide deep frying pan over medium heat. Add the onion and one clove of the garlic and sauté until the onion is tender. Add the tomatoes and tomato paste and bring to a simmer. Add the remaining garlic and simmer over low heat for 30 minutes. Add the herbs, cinnamon, and salt and freshly ground pepper to taste, and continue to simmer another 15 minutes. Remove from the heat and blend together with the cottage cheese in a food processor or a blender. Return to the pan and keep warm while you heat the water for the pasta.

Bring a large pot of water to a rolling boil, add a teaspoon of salt and the pasta. Cook al dente, just until tender to the bite, 5 to 10 minutes, depending on the pasta. Drain and toss with the sauce, and serve at once. Or distribute the pasta among the plates and top each serving with the sauce. Pass the freshly grated Parmesan in a bowl. (Serves 4 to 6.)

Spinach Lasagne.

You can use the tomato sauce below for this, or a good brand of commercial tomato sauce, which you can find in natural foods stores. You need one quart of sauce.

For the tomato sauce:
1 medium onion, chopped   Vitamin A ++
3 cloves garlic, minced or put through a press   Vitamin C ++
1 tablespoon safflower oil
3 pounds tomatoes (canned or fresh),
   seeded and chopped
6 ounces tomato paste
Salt to taste
1 teaspoon oregano
1 teaspoon dried basil (or 1 tablespoon fresh)
½ teaspoon thyme
Pinch of cinnamon
Freshly ground pepper to taste

For the rest of the lasagne:
1 pound low-fat cottage cheese   Protein +++
2 10-ounce packages frozen   Calcium +++
   spinach, thawed   Magnesium ++
Pinch of nutmeg   Complex carbohydrate ++
2 eggs, beaten
Freshly ground pepper to taste
½ pound skim milk mozzarella or
   farmer cheese, sliced thin
1 cup freshly grated Parmesan cheese
12 whole wheat lasagne noodles

First prepare the sauce. Heat the safflower oil in a large, heavy-bottomed frying pan or casserole, and sauté the onion and 2 cloves of the garlic until the onion is tender. Add the tomatoes, tomato paste, and salt, and bring to a simmer. Cover and simmer 30 minutes. Add the remaining garlic, the oregano, basil, and thyme, and simmer, covered, another 30 minutes. Add the cinnamon and freshly ground pepper to taste, and set aside.

Squeeze excess moisture out of the spinach by wrapping in a towel and twisting, and chop fine. Beat the eggs in a bowl and stir in the cottage cheese, spinach, nutmeg, and ground pepper.

Bring a large pot of water to a rolling boil, add a teaspoon of salt, and cook the noodles until just firm to the bite (5 to 10 minutes, depending on the thickness of the noodles). Drain and rinse under cold water. Lay noodles over the sides of the colander so the water will run off as you assemble the lasagne.

Preheat the oven to 350°. Oil a 3- or 4-quart baking dish or casserole. Spread a very thin layer of the tomato sauce on the bottom of the dish and lay 4 noodles across. Top the noodles with ⅓ of the spinach–cottage cheese mixture, spreading it in an even layer over the noodles. Spread ⅓ of the mozzarella or farmer cheese over the spinach mixture, and top with ⅓ of the tomato sauce. Top this with ⅓ of the Parmesan. Repeat the layers two more times: noodles, spinach–cottage cheese mixture, mozzarella or farmer cheese, tomato sauce, and Parmesan.

Bake in the preheated oven for 40 minutes, until bubbling. Serve hot.

Note: This can be made a couple of days in advance and kept in the refrigerator. The tomato sauce will keep for 3 days in the refrigerator, and can be frozen. The lasagne freezes well. (Serves 6 to 8.)

Black Bean Burritos

These can be served hot or cold. They make a great bag lunch. If serving hot, serve the lettuce or alfalfa sprouts and tomatoes on the side.

6 whole wheat flour tortillas
(available in natural foods stores)
2 cups cooked black beans
(see recipe, page 260)
1 teaspoon ground cumin
1 teaspoon chili powder

Complex carbohydrate +++
Protein +++
Calcium ++

    1 teaspoon safflower oil
½ cup grated cheddar or Monterrey
    Jack cheese
    1 cup shredded lettuce or alfalfa
    sprouts
2–3 tomatoes, chopped

If preparing the burritos to be eaten hot, preheat the oven to 325°. Wrap the tortillas in foil and place them in the oven while you prepare the beans.

Drain the beans, retaining about ½ cup of their liquid. Coarsely puree, using the pulse action, in a food processor or blender, along with the cumin and chili powder. Moisten with the bean broth.

Heat the oil in a large nonstick skillet and add the beans. Sauté, stirring, for about 10 minutes.

Remove the tortillas from the oven and spread the refried beans down the center. Top with the cheese and roll up. Heat in the oven for about 15 to 20 minutes, until the cheese melts. Serve with the chopped tomatoes and lettuce on the side. (Serves 6.)

If packing the burritos for a school lunch, spread the beans down the center of the tortillas, then top with cheese, lettuce or sprouts, and tomato. Roll up and wrap tightly in plastic wrap or foil. Refrigerate overnight.

Meatless Chili

2 onions, chopped
4 large cloves garlic, minced or put
    through a press
1 tablespoon safflower oil
2 large carrots, chopped or grated
1 large bell pepper, chopped
2 large cans tomatoes, drained and
    chopped (or 3 pounds fresh ripe
    tomatoes, chopped)
1 small can tomato paste
1 bay leaf
1 tablespoon chili powder
2 teaspoons cumin

Complex carbohydrate ++
Protein ++
Potassium ++
Fiber +

2 dried cayenne peppers (¼ teaspoon
cayenne pepper)
1–2 dried poblano chilis, if available
(optional)
Salt and freshly ground pepper to taste
3 cups cooked red or kidney beans
(may use canned), with ½ cup of their
liquid
1 teaspoon oregano

Heat the safflower oil in a large, heavy-bottomed casserole or soup pot. Add the onions and half the garlic and sauté until the onion begins to soften. Add the carrots and bell pepper and continue to sauté another 3 to 5 minutes, stirring all the while with a wooden spoon.

Add the tomatoes, tomato paste, bay leaf, and spices and bring to a simmer. Crumble in the optional dried poblano pepper and add the remaining garlic. Reduce heat, cover and simmer over very low heat, stirring occasionally, for 30 minutes. Stir in the beans and oregano and continue to cook another 30 minutes. Check from time to time to be sure that the chili doesn't stick. Adjust seasonings, adding salt, pepper, garlic, or cayenne to taste.

Serve with cornbread or corn tortillas, or with whole wheat bread, and a big green salad. (Serves 4.)

Crustless Tofu Quiche

1 tablespoon safflower oil
2 cloves garlic, minced or put
through a press
1 small onion, chopped
1¼ pounds tofu
½ cup plain low-fat yogurt
1 egg (optional)
1 tablespoon whole wheat flour
2 tablespoons soy sauce
1 teaspoon nutritional yeast, or ½
teaspoon yeast extract such as Marmite
or Vegex (see ingredients section)
1 teaspoon sesame tahini

Protein +++
Complex carbohydrate ++
B complex ++

1 teaspoon freshly grated ginger
Juice of ½ lemon
½ teaspoon thyme
Pinch each of cayenne and nutmeg
Freshly ground pepper to taste

Preheat the oven to 350°.

Heat the safflower oil in a frying pan and sauté the onion and garlic until the onion is tender. Set aside.

Combine the remaining ingredients in a blender or food processor and blend until completely smooth. Stir in the onion and garlic.

Oil either a 1½-quart baking dish, a loaf pan, or a 9- or 10-inch tart pan, and pour in the tofu mixture. Smooth the top with a spatula and bake 30 to 40 minutes, until set and the top is beginning to brown. Let sit 10 minutes before serving. This is good hot or cold, and will keep for several days in the refrigerator. It's good for a bag lunch. (Serves 6.)

Homemade Pizza

There is no reason why you shouldn't eat pizza, as long as it's not loaded with cheese and pepperoni or sausage, which are very high in fat. Almost all natural food stores now carry frozen whole wheat pizza crusts, and there are good brands of tomato sauce available too. So in no time you can put together your own healthy versions, topped with whatever vegetables you like. Below are several ways to go about making pizzas, so that even those people who hate to cook won't be deprived of this treat.

For quick whole wheat pizza crust:

2 cups whole wheat or whole wheat pastry flour
½ teaspoon salt
1 teaspoon baking powder
½ teaspoon baking soda
½ cup water, plus 1 or 2 tablespoons more as needed
2 tablespoons vegetable or safflower oil

Complex carbohydrate +++
Protein ++

Mix together the flour, salt, baking powder, and baking soda. Add the water and work in with your hands, then add the oil and work it in (this can also be done in an electric mixer or a food processor). The dough will be stiff and dry. Oil a 10-inch pie pan, pizza pan, or quiche pan. Roll out the dough about ¼ inch thick and line the pan. Since the dough is stiff, this will take some elbow grease. Just keep pounding down with the rolling pin and rolling out until you get a nice flat, round dough. Don't worry if it tears; you can always patch it together. Pinch a nice edge around the top and refrigerate until ready to use. This can also be frozen.

For yeasted pizza crust (2 10-inch crusts):

¾ cup lukewarm water

1 tablespoon active dry yeast

Complex carbohydrate +++
Protein +

1 teaspoon honey

1 teaspoon salt

3 tablespoons safflower oil

2 cups whole wheat or whole wheat pastry flour

Additional flour for kneading, if necessary

Corn meal for the pan

In a large bowl, dissolve the yeast in the water and stir in the honey. Let sit for 10 minutes. Stir in the salt and oil, then fold in 1½ cups of the flour. Place the remaining ½ cup of flour on your kneading surface and turn out the dough. Knead, folding the dough over toward you, then leaning into it, turning the dough a quarter turn and folding and leaning into it again, for 10 minutes. Repeat the fold-lean-turn rhythm, and add flour as necessary to your kneading surface as the dough begins to stick. When the dough is smooth and elastic, form it into a ball, then oil your bowl and place the dough in it seam-side-up first, then seam-side-down. Cover with a damp towel or plastic wrap and place in a warm place to rise for 1 to 1½ hours, until it has doubled in volume.

Punch the dough down and knead again for about a minute. Then divide into two pieces and roll out each piece about ¼ inch thick. Oil two pie pans or pizza pans and dust with cornmeal. Line the pans and pinch a lip around the edge. Cover with plastic and refrigerate or freeze until ready to use. (For this recipe you will only be using one of the crusts, so wrap the second one tightly with plastic or foil, place in a plastic bag, and freeze for a future pizza.)

For the tomato sauce:

1 tablespoon safflower oil	Vitamin A ++

2–3 cloves garlic, minced or put through a press
  2 pounds tomatoes, either fresh or canned, seeded and chopped
  2 tablespoons tomato paste
Salt and freshly ground pepper to taste
  1 teaspoon oregano
  ½ teaspoon thyme
Pinch of cinnamon

Additional toppings:

½ cup grated Parmesan or gruyère cheese	Calcium ++
2 ounces skim milk mozzarella cheese, sliced	Protein +++

  4 ounces tofu, sliced and sprinkled with soy sauce
  1 cup sliced mushrooms, sautéed for 2 minutes in 2 teaspoons safflower oil
  1 onion, sliced in rings
  1 green pepper, sliced in rings
  1 zucchini, thinly sliced and sautèed for 2 minutes in 2 teaspoons safflower oil
Additional garlic, minced or put through a press

Make the crust of your choice. For the tomato sauce, heat the oil in a heavy-bottomed frying pan or casserole and sauté the garlic for about 1 minute. Add the tomatoes and tomato paste and bring to a simmer. Add salt to tàste and cook uncovered for about 30 minutes over medium-low heat, stirring from time to time. Add the oregano and thyme and cook another 15 minutes. Add a pinch of cinnamon and freshly ground pepper to taste. Taste and correct seasonings, adding salt, garlic, or herbs if you wish. Set aside.

If you are using the quick pizza crust, preheat the oven to 450°. If you are using the yeasted pizza crust, preheat the oven to 400° and prebake for 5 minutes, then raise the heat to 450°.

Spread the tomato sauce over the pie crust. Top with the cheese, tofu, and vegetables of your choice. Bake in the preheated oven for 15 minutes, or until the crust is brown and crisp.

Note: You can make this pizza using store-bought tomato sauce and crust, as long as they are reliable products (read the labels). Just assemble as instructed above and top with the vegetables of your choice. Bake as above.

All of these pizzas can be frozen.

Pizza Sandwiches

When you want something like a pizza, but don't feel like going through the hassle of making the crust, use whole-grain bread. Spread with tomato sauce and the toppings of your choice, top with another piece of bread, wrap in aluminum foil, and heat in the oven—or leave open-faced and heat under the broiler without wrapping.

Soft Potato Bean Tacos

Unlike traditional tacos, these are made with tortillas that have been heated but not fried, so they don't have nearly as much fat. They're called "soft tacos" because the tortillas are not crisp. This makes them easier to eat than the usual kind.

1 pound new or boiling potatoes, diced   Protein ++
                                     Complex carbohydrate ++
3 cups cooked black, kidney, or
  pinto beans (may use canned), with their liquid
1 teaspoon chili powder
1 teaspoon ground cumin
1 tablespoon safflower oil
1 small onion, sliced
12 corn tortillas
Salsa Fresca (see recipe, page 258)

Steam the potatoes for 10 minutes, until just tender. Set aside.

Place the beans, with the chili powder, cumin, and ¼ cup of their liquid, in a food processor or blender and blend, using the pulse action, just until slightly pureed. They should still maintain some texture.

Heat the oil in a heavy-bottomed, preferably nonstick skillet and add the onion. Sauté, stirring over medium-high heat, until tender. Add the potatoes and sauté over medium-high heat until they begin to brown. Remove from the skillet and add the beans, and a little more of their liquid if the skillet is very dry. Sauté, stirring over medium heat, for 5 minutes. Remove from the heat and clean the skillet.

Heat the tortillas in the skillet, or steam above boiling water, until flexible and warm. Spread a heaping tablespoon of refried beans down the middle of each and top with a heaping tablespoon of the potato-onion mixture. Roll up the tortilla like an enchilada. Keep warm in a 300° oven while you prepare the rest of the tacos.

Serve warm, with Salsa Fresca. (Makes 12 tacos.)

Salsa Fresca

4 large ripe tomatoes, chopped	Vitamin A ++
½ small onion, minced	
2 tablespoons chopped celantro	
2 serrano or jalapeño peppers, fresh or canned, minced	
2 tablespoons red wine vinegar	
2 tablespoons water	
Salt to taste	

Mix together all the ingredients in a bowl. Chill until ready to serve. This will keep for 2 or 3 days in the refrigerator. (Makes 2 cups.)

Stir-Fried Tofu and Vegetables

1 tablespoon safflower oil	Protein +++
1 onion, sliced	Complex carbohydrate ++
1 clove garlic, minced or put through a press	Vitamin A ++
1 tablespoon grated fresh ginger	Calcium +
¾–1 pound tofu, to taste, diced	Magnesium +
1 tablespoon soy sauce	
1 large carrot, sliced	

1–2 cups regular or Chinese cabbage,
    shredded
  2 tablespoons sesame or sunflower
    seeds
  1 zucchini, sliced (or 1 cup broccoli
    florets)
Water
1–2 additional tablespoons soy sauce
  1 teaspoon vinegar
  1 teaspoon honey
  ¼ cup water
  1 tablespoon cornstarch

Heat the oil in a nonstick skillet and sauté the onion, garlic, and ginger until the onion is tender. Add the tofu and 1 tablespoon soy sauce and sauté, stirring, for 5 minutes. Add the carrot and a couple tablespoons of water. Cook, stirring, for about 5 minutes, and add the cabbage and sesame or sunflower seeds. Cook, stirring another 5 minutes, adding a little water if necessary. Add the zucchini or broccoli and sauté another 5 minutes. Add a little water if necessary, cover, and simmer over medium heat for 5 minutes. Meanwhile, mix together the soy sauce, vinegar, honey, water, and cornstarch in a small bowl. Stir into the tofu-vegetable mixture and continue to cook, stirring, until the tofu and vegetables are glazed. Remove from the heat and serve with hot cooked grains, such as brown rice, bulgur, millet, or couscous. (Serves 4.)

Vegetables and Other Side Dishes

Steamed Artichokes with Tofu Vinaigrette

4 artichokes
1 recipe Tofu Vinaigrette (page 219)

Complex carbohydrate + +
Fiber + +

Wash the artichokes and trim the stems. Cut the very tops off, and, if you want to get rid of the little spikes at the end of the leaves, trim them with the scissors (this isn't necessary if you don't have much time). Place on a steamer above boiling water, cover, and steam 45 minutes, or until the leaves pull away easily.

Meanwhile make the Tofu Vinaigrette. Serve the artichokes hot, room temperature or chilled, and dip the leaves in the Tofu Vinaigrette. (Serves 4.)

Black Beans

2 cups (1 pound) black beans, washed and picked over	Protein +++ Complex carbohydrate ++
6 cups water	
1 tablespoon safflower oil	
1 large onion, chopped	
4 large cloves garlic, minced or put through a press	
Salt to taste	
3–4 tablespoons chopped cilantro	

Wash the beans and carefully pick over to make sure there are no little pebbles disguising themselves as beans. Soak in the 6 cups of water for several hours, or overnight. Drain.

Heat the safflower oil in a large, heavy-bottomed soup pot or Dutch oven and add the onion and two cloves of the garlic. Sauté until the onion is tender and add the drained beans and 6 cups fresh water. Bring to a boil, reduce heat, and cover. Simmer 1 hour. Add the remaining garlic, salt to taste, and the cilantro. Continue to simmer another hour, until the beans are soft and the broth thick and aromatic. Correct seasonings, adding more salt, garlic, or cilantro if you wish, and serve with cornbread, corn tortillas, whole-grain bread, or brown rice. (Serves 4 to 6.)

Bulgur Pilaf

Double the quantity and make Bulgur Pilaf Salad (page 228) for tomorrow's lunch.

1 onion, chopped	Protein + Fiber + Complex carbohydrates +
1 clove garlic, minced or put through a press	
1 tablespoon safflower oil	
1 cup sliced mushrooms	
1 cup bulgur	
¼ teaspoon salt	

2 cups boiling water
Soy sauce and freshly ground pepper to taste

Heat the oil in a lidded nonstick skillet, a wok, or a heavy-bottomed casserole, and add the onion and garlic. Sauté until the onion is tender and add the mushrooms. Continue to sauté another 5 to 10 minutes, until the mushrooms are tender. Add the bulgur and salt, stir together well, then pour in the boiling water. Cover and turn off the heat. Let sit for 20 to 30 minutes without lifting the lid. Then check to see that the bulgur is soft (it should be, but if it isn't, pour on some more boiling water and wait another 15 minutes). Fluff with forks and add soy sauce and freshly ground pepper to taste. Serve hot. (Serves 4.)

Steamed Greens with Vinegar or Lemon Juice

2 pounds collard, mustard, or   Calcium +++
   turnip greens, stems trimmed   Complex carbohydrate ++
   away
1 tablespoon safflower oil
1 clove garlic, minced or put through a press
1–2 tablespoons vinegar or lemon juice,
   to taste
Freshly ground pepper to taste

Wash the greens, and chop them coarsely. Heat a wide heavy frying pan. Add the wet greens and steam in their own liquid, stirring, for about 5 minutes, or until wilted. Remove from the pan and let the liquid in the pan evaporate over medium heat.

Heat the safflower oil in the pan and add the garlic. Sauté for a minute or so, then add the greens. Sauté, stirring, for about 3 minutes, then stir in the vinegar or lemon juice and freshly ground pepper to taste. Serve at once. (This can also be done in advance and reheated). (Serves 4 to 6.)

Mushroom Toasts

4–6 slices toasted whole-grain bread   Complex carbohydrate +++
1 tablespoon safflower oil   Protein ++
½ pound mushrooms, cleaned,   Calcium +
   trimmed, and sliced

1–2 cloves garlic, minced or put through
   a press
½ teaspoon thyme
½ teaspoon rosemary, crushed
1 teaspoon soy sauce
2 tablespoons dry white wine
Freshly ground pepper to taste
2 tablespoons grated Swiss cheese

In a large, heavy-bottomed frying pan heat the oil and add the mushrooms and garlic. Sauté the mushrooms over medium-high heat for about 10 minutes, stirring. Add the herbs, soy sauce, and white wine, and continue to sauté another 5 to 10 minutes. Add freshly ground pepper to taste.

Heat the broiler.

Place the mushrooms over the toasted bread and sprinkle on the cheese. Place under the broiler just until the cheese melts. Serve at once. (Serves 4 to 6.)

Steamed New Potatoes with Herbs

2 pounds new potatoes, scrubbed
2 teaspoons safflower oil
2 tablespoons chopped fresh parsley
1 tablespoon chopped fresh dill
Salt and freshly ground pepper to taste

Complex carbohydrate + +
Calcium +
Magnesium +
Vitamin A +
Potassium +

Cut the new potatoes in half if they are very large and place in a steamer above boiling water. Steam 15 to 20 minutes, or until tender, and remove from the heat.

Heat the oil in a frying pan and add the potatoes and herbs. Heat through, tossing the potatoes in the pan until they are coated with the oil and herbs. Add salt and freshly ground pepper to taste and serve. (Serves 4 to 6.)

Baked Potatoes with Low-Fat Toppings

4 baking potatoes

Complex carbohydrate +
Potassium +
Calcium +
Vitamin A +

Preheat the oven to 425°. Puncture the potato skins with a fork and bake 40 minutes to an hour, until tender.

Slit the potatoes open and top with the topping of your choice (see below). You can also scoop out the inside of the potato and mash with the topping, then return to the skin and heat through.

Topping 1:

½ cup plain low-fat yogurt	Calcium ++
½ cup low-fat cottage cheese	Protein ++
1 clove garlic	
2 tablespoons chopped chives or green onion tops	

Blend together the yogurt, cottage cheese, and garlic in a food processor or a blender. Stir in the chives or green onion tops.

Topping 2:

½ cup plain low-fat yogurt	Calcium ++
½ cup cottage cheese	Protein ++
¼ cup chopped fresh parsley	Vitamin A +

Blend together the yogurt and cottage cheese in a food processor or a blender and stir in the parsley.

For other toppings: Use the same combination of ½ cup yogurt blended with ½ cup cottage cheese (or use all yogurt), seasoned with your choice of the following:

    1 tablespoon tomato paste plus a pinch of cayenne
1–2 teaspoons Dijon mustard
    1 teaspoon ground cumin
    1 teaspoon curry powder
    1 teaspoon caraway seeds
    1 teaspoon soy sauce

Italian-Style Spinach

2 pounds fresh spinach (or 1 pound frozen)	Complex carbohydrate ++
	Calcium ++
1 tablespoon safflower oil	Magnesium +
1 clove garlic, minced or put through a press	
Salt and freshly ground pepper to taste	

If using fresh spinach, wash thoroughly and remove the stems. Heat a dry frying pan and sauté the spinach, using the liquid on the leaves as moisture, until wilted. Remove from the heat and squeeze dry.

If using frozen spinach, let thaw or cook using the instructions on the package, and squeeze dry.

Heat the oil in a large, preferably nonstick frying pan, and sauté the garlic for about 1 minute. Add the spinach and sauté for about 2 to 3 minutes, stirring. Add salt and freshly ground pepper to taste and serve hot. (Serves 4 to 6.)

Baked Tomatoes

4–6 firm, ripe tomatoes   Potassium ++
  2 cloves garlic, minced   Vitamin C +
  ½ teaspoon thyme
  ½ teaspoon crushed rosemary
Salt and freshly ground pepper to taste

Preheat the oven to 400°. Lightly oil a baking dish.

Cut a shallow cone shape out of the stem end of the tomatoes. Sprinkle the cut part with garlic, thyme, rosemary, and salt and pepper to taste.

Bake the tomatoes for about 15 minutes in the hot oven, just until the skins begin to shrivel. Serve hot. (Serves 4 to 6.)

Desserts

Baked Dishes

Baked Apples

4 tart apples   Magnesium +
½ cup apple juice   Calcium +
Cinnamon and nutmeg to taste   Vitamin C +
 2 teaspoons vanilla extract   Essential fatty acid +
 3 tablespoons raisins
 2 tablespoons sunflower seeds
Plain low-fat yogurt for topping

Preheat the oven to 350°. Lightly butter a baking dish.

Cut a cone-shaped cavity into the stem end of each apple and spoon a tablespoon of apple juice into each one. Sprinkle on cinnamon and nutmeg to taste, and ½ teaspoon vanilla extract, then fill each one with the raisins and sunflower seeds. Add the remaining apple juice to the pan. Bake in the preheated oven until tender, about 45 minutes, basting from time to time with the apple juice in the pan. Serve topped with plain low-fat yogurt. (Serves 4.)

Baked Pears

4–6 pears, peeled, cored, and quartered	Complex carbohydrate ++
½ cup apple juice	Vitamin C ++
Cinnamon and nutmeg to taste	
Plain low-fat yogurt for topping (optional)	

Preheat the oven to 350°.

Place the peeled, cored, and quartered pears in a baking dish and pour in the apple juice. Sprinkle with cinnamon and nutmeg and cover the dish with foil or a lid.

Bake in the preheated oven for 30 minutes, until the pears are soft but not mushy, and aromatic. Serve hot or cool, with a spoonful or two of the apple juice. Top, if you wish, with plain low-fat yogurt. (Serves 4 to 6.)

Apple Crisp

6 tart apples	Vitamin C +
Juice of 1 lemon	Magnesium +
1 teaspoon cinnamon	Fiber +
½ teaspoon nutmeg	
¼ teaspoon cloves	
2 tablespoons sunflower seeds	
1 tablespoon cornstarch dissolved in 2 tablespoons water	
2 teaspoons vanilla	

For the topping:

1½ cups rolled oats	1 teaspoon allspice	Complex
½ cup whole wheat flour	⅓ cup safflower oil	carbohy-
¼ teaspoon salt	⅓ cup honey	drate ++
2 teaspoons cinnamon		

Preheat the oven to 375°. Oil or butter a 2-quart baking dish.

Combine the apples, lemon juice, cinnamon, nutmeg, cloves, sunflower seeds, cornstarch dissolved in water, and vanilla. Spread evenly in the prepared baking dish.

Using a food processor or in a bowl with a wooden spoon, mix together the ingredients for the topping and combine well. Spread evenly over the apple mixture.

Bake in the preheated oven for 30 to 45 minutes, until the top is brown and crisp. Serve warm, topped with plain low-fat yogurt. (Serves 6.)

Peach Cobbler

For the filling:

4 cups sliced peaches	Vitamin C +
2 teaspoons vanilla	
½ teaspoon cinnamon	
Juice of ½ lemon	
1 tablespoon cornstarch or arrowroot	

For the topping:

½ cup whole wheat flour	Protein ++
1 cup corn meal	Complex carbohydrate ++
1 tablespoon baking powder	Calcium ++
¼ teaspoon salt	
2 eggs	
1 cup skim milk or plain low-fat yogurt	
¼ cup honey	
2 tablespoons safflower oil	

For garnish:

½ cup plain low-fat yogurt

Preheat the oven to 350°. Butter a 9 × 13-inch baking dish or a 10- to 12-inch pie pan.

Toss together the peaches, vanilla, and cinnamon. Dissolve the cornstarch or arrowroot in the lemon juice and mix with the peaches.

Sift together the whole wheat flour, corn meal, baking powder, and salt. In a separate bowl beat together the eggs, milk or yogurt, honey, and safflower oil. Fold into the dry ingredients and stir together thoroughly. Do not overbeat; a few lumps are okay.

Spread the peaches in the prepared baking dish. Pour the cornbread topping evenly over the peaches. It will be very runny but it will stay on the surface.

Bake the cobbler in the preheated oven for 30 to 40 minutes, until the top is golden brown and the peaches are bubbling. Remove from the oven, let cool a few minutes, and serve. This is good topped with plain low-fat yogurt. It is also good cold or reheated, for breakfast. (Serves 6 to 8.)

Granola Bars

2 cups granola
2 eggs, beaten
2 tablespoons honey (optional)

Protein ++
Fiber +

Preheat the oven to 325°. Oil a baking sheet or 1½- or 2-quart baking pan.

Mix together the eggs and granola and honey if you wish. Spread evenly in the baking pan, ¼ to ½ inch thick. Don't worry if the mixture doesn't reach the edges of the pan.

Bake in the preheated oven for 20 to 30 minutes, until brown and crisp. Remove from the oven and carefully remove from the pan with a spatula. Cut in squares and cool on a rack. (Makes 12 bars.)

Oatmeal Cookies

½ cup honey (use ¼ cup if you can)
½ cup safflower oil
1 egg
2 teaspoons vanilla
¾ teaspoon cinnamon
½ teaspoon nutmeg
¼ teaspoon ground cloves
¼ teaspoon salt
½ teaspoon baking soda
2½ cups rolled oats
1 cup whole wheat or whole wheat pastry flour
1 cup raisins

Complex carbohydrate ++
Fiber ++
Protein +

Preheat the oven to 350°. Oil baking sheets.

Cream together the honey and oil and beat in the egg and vanilla. Stir in the spices.

Mix together the salt, baking soda, rolled oats, and flour. Stir into the wet ingredients and combine well. (This can be done in a food processor or electric mixer). Stir in the raisins.

Drop by the tablespoonful onto the baking sheets and bake in the preheated oven for 12 to 15 minutes, until beginning to brown. Cool on racks. (Makes 4 dozen cookies.)

Noodle Kugel

This recipe is from *Fast Vegetarian Feasts*, by Martha Rose Shulman. It makes a great breakfast, as well as dessert or snack.

2 eggs	Complex carbohydrate ++
1 egg white	Protein ++
1 cup plain low-fat yogurt	Calcium ++
½ cup low-fat cottage cheese	Fiber +
3 tablespoons mild-flavored honey (or less if you can)	
1 tablespoon lemon juice	
½–1 teaspoon cinnamon, to taste	
¼–½ teaspoon nutmeg, to taste	
1 teaspoon vanilla	
¼ cup currants or raisins	
1 apple, chopped	
¼ pound flat whole wheat noodles or 1 cup whole wheat macaroni.	

Preheat the oven to 325° and lightly butter a 1½- or 2-quart baking dish.

Begin heating a large pot of water for the noodles. In a large bowl, beat the eggs and egg white together with the yogurt, cottage cheese, honey, lemon juice, cinnamon, nutmeg, and vanilla. Stir in the raisins or currants and the apple.

Cook the pasta al dente, just firm to the bite, and drain. Rinse with cold water in a strainer and shake out the excess water. Add to the egg mixture and combine well. Turn into the buttered casserole and cover with foil or a lid.

Bake for 35 to 45 minutes, until firm and a crust has begun

to form around the outside. Remove from the oven and allow to stand for 15 minutes before serving. (Serves 6.)

Millet Raisin Pudding

1 cup raw millet	Complex carbohydrate +
4 cups skim milk (or 2 cups water with 2 cups skim milk)	Calcium ++
¼ teaspoon salt	Fiber +

1 cup raw millet
4 cups skim milk (or 2 cups water with 2 cups skim milk)
¼ teaspoon salt
2 teaspoons vanilla extract
¼ cup honey (use less if you can)
½ teaspoon cinnamon
½ teaspoon nutmeg
½ cup raisins

Complex carbohydrate +
Calcium ++
Fiber +

Preheat the oven to 350°. Combine the millet and milk (or water and milk) in a saucepan and bring to a boil on top of the stove. Remove from the heat at once and stir in the remaining ingredients.

Oil a 2-quart baking dish and fill with the millet mixture. Cover with foil or a lid and bake in the preheated oven for 30 to 40 minutes, until the liquid is absorbed. (Serves 4 to 6.)

Brown Rice Pudding

This is a great way to use up leftover brown rice. It makes a great breakfast as well as dessert or snack.

2 eggs
1 cup skim milk
Pinch of salt
¼ cup honey
1 teaspoon vanilla
1 tablespoon lemon juice
½ teaspoon ground cinnamon
¼ teaspoon nutmeg
¼ cup raisins
2 small apples, cored and chopped
1½ cups cooked brown rice
Plain low-fat yogurt or skim milk for topping

Protein ++
Calcium ++

Preheat the oven to 325° and lightly butter a 1½- or 2-quart baking dish.

Beat the eggs together with the milk, salt, and honey. Stir in the vanilla, lemon juice, spices, raisins, and apples. Fold in the cooked brown rice.

Turn the mixture into the prepared baking dish and bake 50 minutes in the preheated oven, or until set. Serve warm or cool, topped if you wish with plain low-fat yogurt or warm skim milk. (Serves 4.)

Fruit Desserts

Fruit Salads

There are all kinds of combinations of fruits that you can use for fruit salads. What you choose should depend primarily on the season; i.e., what's available. Quantities for fruit salad should range from ½ to 1 fruit per person, or ½ to 1 cup fruit per person, depending on how much fruit you eat during the rest of the day. If you have already eaten three pieces of fruit during the course of the day, then eat ½ cup or ½ fruit at night.

In addition to the variety of fruits you can use for a fruit salad, there are a number of ways you can dress them up. Below are suggestions for the salads and garnishes.

Blueberries and peaches or nectarines

Blueberries and oranges

Oranges, grapefruit, and pears

Apples, bananas, and pears

Pineapples, strawberries, and oranges

Assorted melon balls

Cantaloupe and berries

Melon, strawberry, and pineapple

Papaya and strawberries

Mangoes and strawberries

Kiwi, strawberries, and oranges

Fresh figs and grapes

Mixed berries

Suggested Garnishes (for a fruit salad for 4 to 6 people):

Fresh chopped mint

2–3 tablespoons raisins or currants

2–3 tablespoons sunflower seeds

2–3 tablespoons chopped or slivered almonds

Freshly squeezed lemon, lime, or orange juice

Fresh or powdered ginger

Ground cinnamon or nutmeg

3 tablespoons grated unsweetened coconut

Allowing for variations depending on the ingredients you choose, fruit salads provide you with vitamin C (++), complex carbohydrate (++), and fiber (+[++]).

Winter Fruit Ambrosia

2 oranges, peeled, white pith removed, and cut in sections	Vitamin C ++
	Complex carbohydrate ++
1 grapefruit, peeled, white pith removed, cut in sections	Fiber +
¼ cup chopped dates or figs	
2 tablespoons chopped or slivered almonds	
1 apple, cored and chopped	
Juice of ½ lime	
1 tablespoon honey (optional)	
¼ cup unsweetened grated coconut	

Toss together the oranges, grapefruit, dates or figs, apple, and almonds. Stir together the lime juice and honey and toss with the fruit. Add the coconut, toss once more, and serve. (Serves 4 to 6.)

Dried Fruit Compote with Yogurt

1 cup dried apricots	Vitamin C ++
1 cup prunes	Fiber ++
¼ cup raisins	Calcium +
½ cup chopped dried pears or peaches	
1 stick cinnamon	

    4 cups water
    1 cup plain low-fat yogurt

Place the dried fruit and cinnamon stick in a saucepan and cover with the water. Bring to a simmer and simmer 30 minutes.

Serve topped with plain low-fat yogurt. (Serves 4 to 6.)

Apples with Lime Juice

    4–6 apples, cored and sliced   Vitamin C ++
    Juice of 2 limes

Toss the sliced apples with the lime juice and refrigerate until ready to serve. (Serves 4 to 6.)

Poached Bananas

    2 cups apple juice   Vitamin C +
    Juice of ½ lemon   Calcium ++
    ¼ cup raisins   Complex carbohydrate ++
    1 tablespoon vanilla extract
    1 3-inch stick of cinnamon
    3 ripe but firm bananas
    Freshly grated nutmeg to taste
    ½ cup plain low-fat yogurt

Combine the apple juice, lemon juice, raisins, vanilla, and cinnamon in a 4- or 5-quart saucepan and bring to a simmer. Simmer 5 minutes. Peel the bananas and slice into the mixture. Simmer another 10 minutes. Sprinkle on fresh nutmeg and serve, garnishing each serving with a dollop of yogurt. The bananas can be served hot, warm, or at room temperature. The leftovers (if there are any) are good on hot cereal, with additional yogurt. (Serves 4 to 6.)

Berries with Yogurt

    2½ cups fresh or frozen (without sugar)   Vitamin C ++
        berries, such as blueberries, raspberries,   Calcium ++
        boysenberries, blackberries, or strawberries

Juice of ½ lemon
 1 tablespoon honey (optional)
 2 cups plain low-fat yogurt

Using the back of a spoon, a mixer, or a food processor, mash
1 cup of the berries along with the lemon juice and honey. Stir
together the mashed berries with the remaining berries and the
yogurt, and serve. Or place the yogurt in individual bowls and
top with the berry mixture. (Serves 4.)

Oranges with Figs

3–4 oranges, peeled, white pith cut away, and   Vitamin C ++
      cut into sections   Fiber ++
 ½ cup chopped dried figs
 ½ teaspoon cinnamon

Toss together the oranges, figs, and cinnamon and serve, or
refrigerate and serve cold. (Serves 4 to 6.)

Pear Compote

3 cups apple juice   Vitamin C ++
 2 teaspoons vanilla
Juice of 1 lemon
 1 stick cinnamon (or ½ teaspoon powdered cinnamon)
 3 tablespoons raisins
 6 firm, ripe pears
 ½ cup plain low-fat yogurt, for topping (optional)

Combine the apple juice, vanilla, lemon juice, cinnamon,
and raisins in a saucepan large enough to accommodate the
pears. Bring to a simmer and simmer 5 minutes.

Peel, core, and quarter the pears and drop immediately into
the simmering apple juice. Poach in the juice for 8 to 10 minutes. Remove from the heat. Serve warm or cooled, spooning the
liquid over the pears and topping if you wish with a spoonful of
plain low-fat yogurt. (Serves 6.)

Frozen Desserts

Banana Yogurt Ice Cream

This is as satisfying as ice cream. You need to remember to freeze the bananas in advance, and you must have a food processor to do it. If you like ice cream, it's worth investing in a food processor just for this.

4 bananas, peeled and frozen	Potassium ++
1 cup plain low-fat yogurt	Calcium ++
2–3 teaspoons vanilla extract	
Nutmeg to taste	

Cut the frozen bananas into chunks and place in the food processor with the remaining ingredients. Using the start-stop action, blend together until you have a smooth mixture. From time to time you might have to remove pieces of banana from the blades. Make sure you use the start-stop action of your food processor and not the continuous action, or your ice cream will become too liquid.

When the mixture is smooth, serve at once. (Serves 4.)

Yogurt Ice Pops

2 cups plain low-fat yogurt	Calcium ++
½ cup Apple Puree (page 205) or 1 small can	Vitamin C +
orange juice concentrate	
2 teaspoons honey	
2 teaspoons vanilla	

Blend together all the ingredients and pour into paper cups. Cover each cup with foil and insert ice pop sticks into the middle of each one. (You can also use ice pop molds.)

Freeze for several hours. (Serves 4 to 6.)

Frozen Apple Yogurt

See recipe for Yogurt Ice Pops, above. Use version with Apple Puree. You can freeze this in ice pop molds or in a container. Soften for 30 minutes in the refrigerator before eating. (Serves 4.)

Orange Ice

4 cups orange juice (can be from   Vitamin C + +
   unsweetened concentrate)

Place the orange juice in an ice cream maker or sherbet maker and process until frozen.

You can make this without an ice cream maker by freezing the juice in ice-cube trays (without the separators) and breaking it up after 1 hour in the freezer in a food processor or electric mixer. Return to the freezer and freeze until just about frozen solid. Break up once more before serving. (Serves 4 to 6.)

Strawberry or Raspberry Ice

4 cups frozen strawberries or raspberries   Vitamin C +
1 tablespoon honey   Calcium + +
1 tablespoon lemon juice
½ teaspoon ground cinnamon
1 cup plain low-fat yogurt

Place all the ingredients in a food processor and pulse on and off until the berries are mashed. Then puree until the mixture is smooth. Serve at once, or store in the freezer.

Note: When you store this in the freezer it will freeze solid. Let soften in the refrigerator for 30 minutes before serving. You can also make ice pops by freezing the mixture in ice pop molds or paper cups. (Serves 4.)

Appendix I: Summary Chart of Nutrients

Nutrients	Importance	Deficiency Symptoms	RDA*	Toxicity Level
Carbohydrate	Provides energy for body functions and muscular exertions. Assists in digestion and assimilation of foods.	Loss of energy. Fatigue. Excessive protein breakdown. Disturbed balance of water, sodium, potassium, and chloride.		Intake should not exceed what is needed to maintain desirable weight.
Fat	Provides energy. Acts as a carrier for fat-soluble vitamins A, D, E, and K. Supplies essential fatty acids needed for growth, health, and smooth skin.	Eczema or skin disorders. Retarded growth	At least 15% of total calories, but no more than 25% of total calories.	Intake should not exceed what is needed to maintain desirable weight.
Protein	Is necessary for growth and development. Acts in formation of hormones, enzymes, and antibodies.	Fatigue. Loss of appetite. Diarrhea and vomiting. Stunted growth. Edema.	45–50 g high-quality protein.	Intake should not exceed what is needed to maintain desirable weight.

	Functions	Deficiency Symptoms	Recommended Dietary Allowance*	Toxicity
VITAMINS				
Vitamin A	Maintains acid-alkali balance. Is source of heat and energy. Is necessary for growth and repair of body tissues. Is important to health of the eyes. Fights bacteria and infection. Maintains healthy epithelial tissue. Aids in bone and teeth formation.	Night blindness. Rough, dry, scaly skin. Increased susceptibility to infections. Frequent fatigue, insomnia, depression. Loss of smell and appetite. Lusterless hair. Brittle nails. Inflamed eyelids.	Infants: 1,400–2,000 IU Children: 2,000–4,000 IU Adults: 4,000–5,000 IU	50,000 to 100,000 IU may be toxic if there is no deficiency and if used daily more than 4–8 weeks.
Vitamin B complex	Is necessary for carbohydrate, fat, and protein metabolism. Helps functioning of the nervous system. Helps maintain muscle tone in the gastrointestinal tract. Maintains health of skin, hair, eyes, mouth, and liver.	Dry, rough, cracked skin. Acne. Dull, dry, or gray hair. Fatigue. Poor appetite. Gastrointestinal tract disorders.	See individual B vitamins	See individual B vitamins; relatively nontoxic.

* Recommended Dietary Allowance

From Nutrition Search, Inc., *Nutrition Almanac*, 2nd ed., McGraw-Hill, New York, 1984. Used by permission.

Nutrients	Importance	Deficiency Symptoms	RDA*	Toxicity Level
Vitamin B₁ (Thiamine)	Is necessary for carbohydrate metabolism. Helps maintain healthy nervous system. Stabilizes the appetite. Stimulates growth and good muscle tone.	Gastrointestinal problems. Fatigue. Loss of appetite. Nerve disorders. Heart disorders. Poor impulse control.	Infants: 0.3–0.5 mg. Children: 0.7–1.2 mg. Men: 1.4 mg. Women: 1.0 mg. Extra needed if on poor diet or with use of alcohol.	No known oral toxicity.
Vitamin B₂ (Riboflavin)	Is necessary for carbohydrate, fat, and protein metabolism. Aids in formation of antibodies and red blood cells. Maintains cell respiration.	Eye problems. Cracks and sores in mouth. Dermatitis. Retarded growth. Digestive disturbances.	Infants: 0.4–0.6 mg. Children: 0.8–1.4 mg. Men: 1.6 mg. Women: 1.2 mg. Extra needed if artificial light used.	No known oral toxicity.
Niacin (B₃, Nicotinic acid, Niacinamide)	Is necessary for carbohydrate, fat, and protein metabolism. Helps maintain health of skin, tongue, and digestive system.	Dermatitis. Nervous disorders. Headaches. Insomnia. Bad breath. Digestive disturbances.	Infants: 6–8 mg. Children: 9–16 mg. Men: 16 mg. Women: 13 mg.	100–300 mg nicotinic acid orally may produce flushing in some individuals.

Pantothenic acid (B₅)	Aids in formation of some fats. Participates in the release of energy from carbohydrates, fats, and proteins. Aids in the utilization of some vitamins. Improves body's resistance to stress.	Sore mouth and gums. Vomiting. Restlessness. Increased susceptibility to infection. Gastrointestinal disturbances. Depression. Fatigue.	Infants: 2–3 mg Children: 3–7 mg Adults: 5–10 mg	500–1,000 mg per day is still safe as treatment for allergy.
Vitamin B₆ (Pyridoxine)	Is necessary for carbohydrate, fat, and protein metabolism. Aids in formation of antibodies. Helps maintain balance of sodium and phosphorus.	Anemia. Mouth disorders. Nervousness. Muscular weakness. Dermatitis. Dandruff. Water retention.	Infants: 0.3–0.6 mg Children: 0.9–1.8 mg Men: 2.2 mg Women: 2 mg	Toxicity possible above 500 mg per day. Women do better at 25–50 mg per day.
Vitamin B₁₂	Is essential for normal formation of blood cells. Is necessary for carbohydrate, fat, and protein metabolism. Maintains healthy nervous system.	Pernicious anemia. Brain damage. Nervousness. Neuritis.	Infants: 0.5–1.5 mcg Children: 2–3 mcg Adults: 3 mcg	No known oral toxicity even with intake as high as 600–1,200 mcg.

* Recommended Dietary Allowance

Nutrients	Importance	Deficiency Symptoms	RDA*	Toxicity Level
Folic acid (Folacin)	Is important in red blood cell formation. Aids metabolism of proteins. Is necessary for growth and division of body cells.	Poor growth. Gastrointestinal disorders. Anemia. Poor memory.	Infants: 0.03–0.045 mg Children: 0.1–0.4 mg Adults: 0.4 mg	No toxic effects
Vitamin C	Maintains collagen. Helps heal wounds, scar tissue, and fractures. Gives strength to blood vessels. May provide resistance to infections. Aids in absorption of iron.	Bleeding gums. Swollen or painful joints. Slow-healing wounds and fractures. Bruising. Nosebleeds. Impaired digestion.	Infants: 35 mg Children: 45–50 mg Adults: 60 mg	Essentially nontoxic. Large doses, 10,000 to 20,000 mg, may soften bowel movements.
Vitamin D	Improves absorption and utilization of calcium and phosphorus required for bone formation. Maintains stable nervous system and normal heart action.	Poor bone and tooth formation. Softening of bones and teeth. Inadequate absorption of calcium. Retention of phosphorus in kidney.	Infants, children, and adults, 400 IU	Doses over 1,000–2,000 IU daily considered potentially toxic.
Vitamin E	Protects fat-soluble vitamins. Protects red blood cells. Is essential in cellular respiration. Inhibits coagulation of blood by preventing blood clots.	Rupture of red blood cells. Muscular wasting. Abnormal fat deposits in muscles.	Infants: 4–6 IU Children: 7–12 IU Men: 15 IU Women: 12 IU	Essentially nontoxic. 4,000–30,000 IU of tocopherol for prolonged periods produces side effects in some persons.

Vitamin K	Is necessary for formation of prothrombin; is needed for blood coagulation.	Lack of prothrombin, increasing the tendency to hemorrhage.	Infants: 12–20 mcg Children: 15–100 mcg Adults: 300–500 mcg No RDA*	Menadione (synthetic vitamin K) may have side effects.
Bioflavonoids (Vitamin P)	Help increase strength of capillaries.	Tendency to bleed and bruise easily.	No RDA	No known toxicity.
Unsaturated fatty acids	Are important for respiration of vital organs. Help maintain resilience and lubrication of cells. Help regulate blood coagulation. Are essential for normal glandular activity.	Brittle, lusterless hair. Brittle nails. Dandruff. Diarrhea. Varicose veins.	No RDA, 10% of total calories	None known, but best to keep them below total of caloric intake.
Saturated fatty acids			No RDA, 10% of total calories	None known, but best to keep them below 20% of total calorie intake.
MINERALS Calcium	Sustains development and maintenance of strong bones and teeth. Assists normal blood clotting, muscle action, nerve function, and heart function.	Tetany, Softening bones. Back and leg pains. Brittle bones. Insomnia. Irritability. Depression.	Infants: 360–540 mg Children: 800–1,200 mg Adults: 800 mg	Excessive intakes of calcium may have side effects in certain persons.

* Recommended Dietary Allowance

Nutrients	Importance	Deficiency Symptoms	RDA*	Toxicity Level
Chlorine	Regulates acid-base balance. Maintains osmotic pressure. Stimulates production of hydrochloric acid. Helps maintain joints and tendons.	Loss of hair and teeth. Poor muscular contractibility. Impaired digestion	No RDA	Daily intake of 14–28 g of salt (sodium chloride) is considered excessive. Excess intake of chlorine may have adverse effects. No known toxicity.
Chromium	Stimulates enzymes in metabolism of energy and synthesis of fatty acids, cholesterol, and protein. Increases effectiveness of insulin.	Depressed growth rate. Glucose intolerance in diabetics. Atherosclerosis.	Infants: 0.01–0.06 mg Children: 0.02–0.2 mg Adults: 0.05–0.2 mg	
Copper	Aids in formation of red blood cells. Is part of many enzymes. Works with vitamin C to form elastin.	General weakness. Impaired respiration. Skin sores.	Infants: 0.5–1 mg Children: 1–3 mg Adults: 2–3 mg	Excessive intakes may have side effects.
Fluorine (Fluoride)	May reduce tooth decay by discouraging the growth of acid-forming bacteria.	Tooth decay.	Infants: 0.1–1 mg Children: 0.5–2.5 mg Adults: 1.5–4 mg	Excessive intake of fluoride may have side effects in some persons.
Iodide	Is essential part of the hormone thyroxine. Is necessary for the	Enlarged thyroid gland. Dry skin and hair. Loss of physical	Infants: 40–50 mcg Children: 70–150 mcg Adults: 150 mcg	Up to 1,000 mcg daily produced no toxic effects in persons

	Functions	Deficiency Symptoms	RDA*	Toxicity
	prevention of goiter. Regulates production of energy and rate of metabolism. Promotes growth.	and mental vigor. Cretinism in children born to iodine-deficient mothers.		with a normal thyroid.**
Iron	Is necessary for hemoglobin and myoglobin formation. Helps in protein metabolism. Promotes growth.	Weakness. Paleness of skin. Constipation. Anemia.	Infants: 10–15 mg Children: 15–18 mg Men: 10 mg Women: 18 mg	Excessive intake may be toxic.
Magnesium	Acts as a catalyst in the utilization of carbohydrates, fats, protein, calcium, phosphorus, and possibly potassium.	Nervousness. Muscular excitability. Tremors. Depression.	Infants: 50–70 mg Children: 150–300 mg Adults: 500 to 1000 mg may be a better amount.	More than 2,000 mg daily may be toxic in certain individuals.
Manganese	Is enzyme activator. Plays a part in carbohydrate and fat production. Is necessary for normal skeletal development. Maintains sex-hormone production.	Paralysis. Convulsions. Dizziness. Ataxia. Blindness and deafness in infants. Diabetes. Loss of hearing.	Infants: 0.5–1 mg Children: 1–5 mg Adults: 2.5–5 mg	Excessive intake may have side effects in certain persons.

* Recommended Dietary Allowance

** Robert S. Goodhart and Maurice E. Shils, *Modern Nutrition in Health and Disease*, 5th ed. (Philadelphia: Lea & Febiger, 1973), p. 365.

Nutrients	Importance	Deficiency Symptoms	RDA*	Toxicity Level
Phosphorus	Works with calcium to build bones and teeth. Utilizes carbohydrates, fats, and proteins. Stimulates muscular contraction.	Loss of weight and appetite. Irregular breathing. Pyorrhea. Fatigue. Nervous disorders.	Infants: 240–360 mg Children: 800–1,200 mg Adults: 800 mg	No known toxicity.
Potassium	Works to control activity of heart muscles, nervous system, and kidneys	Poor reflexes. Respiratory failure. Cardiac arrest. Nervous disorders. Constipation. Irregular pulse. Insomnia.	Infants: 350–1,275 mg Children: 550–4,575 mg Adults: 1,875–5,625 mg	No known toxicity.
Selenium	Works with vitamin E. Preserves tissue elasticity.	Premature aging.	Infants: 0.01–0.06 mg Children: 0.02–0.2 mg Adults: 0.05–0.2 mg	Excessive intake may be toxic.
Sodium	Maintains normal fluid levels in cells. Maintains health of the nervous, muscular, blood, and lymph systems.	Muscle weakness. Muscle shrinkage. Nausea. Loss of appetite. Intestinal gas.	Infants: 115–750 mg Children: 325–2,700 mg Adults: 1,100–3,300 mg	Excessive sodium intake may have adverse effects. Intake of 14–28 g of sodium chloride (salt) is considered excessive.

Sulfur	Is part of amino acids. Is essential for formation of body tissues. Is part of the B vitamins. Plays a part in tissue respiration. Is necessary for collagen synthesis.	Possibly sluggishness and fatigue.	The RDA of protein supplies sufficient amounts of sulfur.	Excessive intake of sulfur may be toxic.
Zinc	Is component of insulin and male reproductive fluid. Aids in digestion and metabolism of phosphorus. Aids in healing process.	Retarded growth. Delayed sexual maturity. Prolonged heating of wounds. Stretch marks. Irregular menses. Diabetes. Loss of taste and appetite.	Infants: 3–5 mg Children: 10–15 mg Adults: 15 mg	Relatively nontoxic. Excessive intake may have side effects.

* Recommended Dietary Allowance

Appendix II: Nutrients That Function Together·

When nutrients are taken in supplemental form, they function best when taken together in particular combinations. Some nutrients are so closely interrelated that their effectiveness in the body is markedly improved when they are taken together with other nutrients. Minerals are especially important in aiding the effectiveness of specific vitamins.

For example, if one is suffering from athlete's foot, vitamin A is recommended as a treatment. Vitamin A can be utilized more effectively within the body when taken with the B-complex vitamins, and vitamins C, D, E, and unsaturated fatty acids. Calcium, phosphorus, and zinc are also recommended to increase the effectiveness of vitamin A.

The following chart provides a basic guide to nutrients that function best when taken together.

A. VITAMINS

1. VITAMIN A IS MORE EFFECTIVE WHEN TAKEN WITH

Vitamin B complex Choline	Helps preserve stored vitamin A.
Vitamin C	Helps protect against toxic effects of vitamin A.
	Helps prevent oxidation.
Vitamin D	1 part vitamin D to 10 parts vitamin A.

From Nutrition Search, Inc., *Nutrition Almanac*, 2nd ed., McGraw-Hill, New York, 1984. Used by permission.

Vitamin E   Acts as an antioxidant.
Unsaturated fatty acids
Calcium
Phosphorus
Zinc   Helps in the absorption of vitamin A.

VITAMIN A ANTAGONISTS

Air pollution
Alcohol
Arsenicals
Aspirin
Corticosteroid drugs
(such as prednisone
and cortisone)
Dicumarol
Mineral oil
Nitrates
Phenobarbital
Thyroid

2. VITAMIN B COMPLEX IS MORE EFFECTIVE WHEN TAKEN WITH
Vitamin C
Vitamin E
Calcium
Phosphorus

VITAMIN B COMPLEX ANTAGONISTS

Alcohol
Antibiotics
Aspirin
Corticosteroid drugs
Diuretics

3. VITAMIN B_1 (THIAMINE) IS MORE EFFECTIVE WHEN TAKEN WITH
Vitamin B complex
Vitamin B_2 (riboflavin)
Folic acid
Niacin
Vitamin C   Helps protect against oxidation.
Vitamin E
Manganese
Sulfur

VITAMIN B$_1$ ANTAGONISTS

Alcohol

Antibiotics

Excess sugar

4. VITAMIN B$_2$ (RIBOVLAVIN) IS MORE EFFECTIVE WHEN TAKEN WITH

Vitamin B complex

Vitamin B$_6$ Vitamin B$_2$ and vitamin B$_6$ doses should usually be about the same.

Niacin

Vitamin C   Helps protect against oxidation.

VITAMIN B$_2$ ANTAGONISTS

Alcohol

Antibiotics

Oral contraceptives

5. NIACIN (B$_3$) IS MORE EFFECTIVE WHEN TAKEN WITH

Vitamin B complex

Vitamin B$_1$ (thiamine)

Vitamin B$_2$ (riboflavin)

Vitamin C   Helps protect against oxidation.

NIACIN ANTAGONISTS

Alcohol

Antibiotics

Excess sugar

6. PANTOTHENIC ACID (B$_5$) IS MORE EFFECTIVE WHEN TAKEN WITH

Vitamin B complex

Vitamin B$_6$ (pyridoxine)

Vitamin B$_{12}$

Biotin   Aids in the absorption of pantothenic acid.

Folic acid   Aids in the absorption of pantothenic acid.

Vitamin C   Helps protect against oxidation.

Calcium

Sulfur

PANTOTHENIC ACID ANTAGONISTS

Aspirin

Methylbromide (an insecticide fumigant for some foods)

7. **VITAMIN B_6 (PYRIDOXINE) IS MORE EFFECTIVE WHEN TAKEN WITH**

Vitamin B complex

Vitamin B_1 (thiamine)   Vitamin B_1 and vitamin B_6 doses should usually be about the same.

Vitamin B_2 (riboflavin)   Vitamin B_2 and vitamin B_6 doses should usually be about the same.

Pantothenic acid

Vitamin C

Magnesium

Potassium

Linoleic acid

Sodium

VITAMIN B_6 ANTAGONISTS

Cortisone

Estrogen

Oral contraceptives

8. **VITAMIN B_{12} IS MORE EFFECTIVE WHEN TAKEN WITH**

Vitamin B complex

Vitamin B_6 (pyridoxine) Helps increase absorption of vitamin B_{12}.

Choline

Folic acid

Inositol

Vitamin C   Helps increase absorption of vitamin B_{12}.

Calcium

Iron   Helps increase absorption of vitamin B_{12}.

Potassium

Sodium

VITAMIN B_{12} ANTAGONISTS

Dilantin

Oral contraceptives

9. **PANGAMIC ACID (B_{15}) IS MORE EFFECTIVE WHEN TAKEN WITH**

Vitamin B complex

Vitamin C

Vitamin E

10. **FOLIC ACID IS MORE EFFECTIVE WHEN TAKEN WITH**

Vitamin B complex

Vitamin B_{12}

Biotin
Pantothenic acid
Vitamin C   Helps protect against oxidation.

FOLIC ACID ANTAGONISTS

Alcohol
Anticonvulsants
Oral contraceptives
Phenobarbital

11. VITAMIN C IS MORE EFFECTIVE WHEN TAKEN WITH
All vitamins and miner-
    als
Bioflavonoids
Calcium   Helps body utilize vitamin C.
Magnesium   Helps body utilize vitamin C.

VITAMIN C ANTAGONISTS

Alcohol
Antibiotics
Antihistamines
Aspirin
Baking soda
Barbiturates
Cortisone
DDT
Estrogen
Oral contraceptives
Petroleum
Smoking
Sulfa drugs

12. VITAMIN D IS MORE EFFECTIVE WHEN TAKEN WITH
Vitamin A   10 parts vitamin A to 1 part vitamin D.
Choline   Helps to prevent toxicity.
Vitamin C   Helps to prevent toxicity.
Unsaturated fatty acids
Calcium
Phosphorus

VITAMIN D ANTAGONISTS

Alcohol

Corticosteroid drugs
Oral contraceptives
Dilantin

13. VITAMIN E IS MORE EFFECTIVE WHEN TAKEN WITH

Vitamin A
Vitamin B complex
Vitamin B$_1$ (thiamine)
Inositol   Helps body utilize vitamin E.
Vitamin C   Helps protect against oxidation.
Unsaturated fatty acids
Manganese   Helps body utilize vitamin E.
Selenium

VITAMIN E ANTAGONISTS

Air pollution
Antibiotics
Chlorine
Hypolipidemic drugs
Inorganic iron
Mineral oil
Oral contraceptives
Rancid fats and oils

UNSATURATED FATTY ACIDS ARE MORE EFFECTIVE WHEN
TAKEN WITH

Vitamin A
Vitamin C
Vitamin D
Vitamin E   Helps prevent oxidation and depletion.
Phosphorus

14. VITAMIN K IS MORE EFFECTIVE WHEN TAKEN WITH
No information is available at this time.

VITAMIN K ANTAGONISTS

Air pollution
Antibiotics
Anticoagulants
Mineral oil
Radiation
Rancid oils and fats

15. BIOFLAVONOIDS (VITAMIN P) ARE MORE EFFECTIVE WHEN TAKEN WITH

Vitamin C

B. MINERALS

1. CALCIUM IS MORE EFFECTIVE WHEN TAKEN WITH

Vitamin A	Aids in absorption.
Vitamin C	Aids in absorption.
Vitamin D	Helps in the reabsorption of calcium in kidney tubules and in the retention and utilization of calcium.
Unsaturated fatty acids	Helps make calcium available to tissues.
Iron	Aids in absorption.
Magnesium	2 parts calcium to 1 part magnesium.
Manganese	
Phosphorus	
Hydrochloric acid	

CALCIUM ANTAGONISTS

Aspirin
Corticosteroid drugs
Thyroid

2. CHLORINE IS MORE EFFECTIVE WHEN TAKEN WITH

No information is available at this time.

3. COPPER IS MORE EFFECTIVE WHEN TAKEN WITH

Cobalt
Iron
Zinc

4. FLUORINE IS MORE EFFECTIVE WHEN TAKEN WITH

No information is available at this time.

5. IODINE IS MORE EFFECTIVE WHEN TAKEN WITH

No information is available at this time.

6. IRON IS MORE EFFECTIVE WHEN TAKEN WITH

Vitamin B_{12}	Helps iron function in the body.
Folic acid	
Vitamin C	Aids in absorption.
Calcium	
Cobalt	

Copper
Phosphorus
Hydrochloric acid   Needed for assimilation of iron.
IRON ANTAGONISTS

Antacids
Aspirin
EDTA (a food preserva-
tive)
Vitamin E

7. MAGNESIUM IS MORE EFFECTIVE WHEN TAKEN WITH
Vitamin B$_6$
Vitamin C
Vitamin D
Calcium   1 part magnesium to 2 parts calcium.
Phosphorus
Protein
MAGNESIUM ANTAGONISTS

Alcohol
Corticosteroid drugs
Diuretics

8. MANGANESE IS MORE EFFECTIVE WHEN TAKEN WITH
Vitamin B$_1$ (thiamine)
Vitamin E
Calcium
Phosphorus
MANGANESE ANTAGONISTS

Antibiotics

9. PHOSPHORUS IS MORE EFFECTIVE WHEN TAKEN WITH
Vitamin A
Vitamin D
Unsaturated fatty acids
Calcium   1 part phosphorus to 2.5 parts calcium.
Iron
Manganese
Protein
PHOSPHORUS ANTAGONISTS

Alcohol

Antacids
Aspirin
Corticosteroid drugs
Diuretics
Thyroid

10. POTASSIUM IS MORE EFFECTIVE WHEN TAKEN WITH
Vitamin B_6
Sodium

POTASSIUM ANTAGONISTS

Aspirin
Corticosteroid drugs
Diuretics
Sodium

11. SELENIUM IS MORE EFFECTIVE WHEN TAKEN WITH
Vitamin E

12. SULFUR IS MORE EFFECTIVE WHEN TAKEN WITH
Vitamin B complex
Vitamin B_1 (thiamine)
Biotin
Pantothenic acid

13. ZINC IS MORE EFFECTIVE WHEN TAKEN WITH
Vitamin A
Vitamin B_6
Vitamin E
Calcium
Copper
Phosphorus

ZINC ANTAGONISTS

Alcohol
Chelating compounds
(use to remove excess
copper)
Corticosteroid drugs
Diuretics
Oral contraceptives

Bibliography and Suggested Reading

Baily, Covert. *Fit or Fat?* Boston: Houghton Mifflin Company, 1978.

Bell, Ruth, and co-authors. *Changing Bodies, Changing Lives.* New York: Random House, 1980.

Bennet, William, M.D., and Gurin, Joel. *The Dieter's Dilemma (Eating Less and Weighing More).* New York: Basic Books, 1982.

Brody, Jane. *Jane Brody's Nutrition Book.* New York: Bantam Books, 1982.

Burum, Linda. *The Junk Food Alternative.* San Francisco: 101 Productions, 1981.

Haas, Dr. Robert. *Eat to Win: The Sport Nutrition Bible.* New York: Rawson Associates, 1983.

McEntire, Patricia. *Mommy, I'm Hungry.* Sacramento: Cougar Books, 1982.

Nutrition Search, Inc. (John D. Kirschmann, Director, Lavon J. Dunne, Co-author). *Nutrition Almanac* (second edition). New York: McGraw-Hill Book Company, 1984.

Olsen, Laurie. *Food Fight: A Report on Teen-agers' Eating Habits and Nutritional Status.* Oakland, Calif.: Citizens Policy Center, 1984.

Rosenzweig, Sandra. *Sportsfitness for Women.* New York: Harper & Row, 1982.

Warner, Penny. *Healthy Snacks for Kids.* Concord, Ca.: Nitty Gritty Productions, 1983.

General Index

Recipe Index

About the Author

Dr. Lendon Smith has been practicing pediatrics since 1951. During most of his practice he has particularly emphasized nutritional counseling for parents. Dr. Smith is former Clinical Professor of Pediatrics at the University of Oregon Medical School and a member of the American Academy of Pediatrics. He first became a favorite of television viewers for his show *The Children's Doctor*—also the title of his first book—and won an Emmy for his television documentary *My Mom's Having a Baby*. Dr. Smith is a frequent guest on the major network television shows and is the author of the best-selling *Improving Your Child's Behavior Chemistry*, *Feed Your Kids Right*, *Foods for Healthy Kids*, *Feed Yourself Right*, and *Dr. Lendon Smith's Low-Stress Diet*. Dr. Smith and his wife live in Portland, Oregon.

Catalog

If you are interested in a list of fine Paperback
books, covering a wide range of subjects
and interests, send your name and address,
requesting your free catalog, to:

McGraw-Hill Paperbacks
1221 Avenue of Americas
New York, N.Y. 10020